Supporting People Living with Dementia in Black, Asian and Minority Ethnic Communities

of related interest

Dementia, Culture and Ethnicity
Issues for All
Edited by Julia Botsford and Karen Harrison Dening
Foreword by Alistair Burns
ISBN 978 1 84905 486 7
eISBN 978 0 85700 881 7

Essentials of Dementia
Everything You Really Need to Know for Working in Dementia Care
Dr Shibley Rahman and Professor Rob Howard
Forewords by Karen Harrison Dening and Kate Swaffer
ISBN 978 1 78592 397 5
eISBN 978 1 78450 754 1

Will I Still Be Me?
Finding a Continuing Sense of Self in the Lived Experience of Dementia
Christine Bryden
ISBN 978 1 78592 555 9
eISBN 978 1 78450 950 7

A Pocket Guide to Understanding Alzheimer's Disease and Other Dementias, Second Edition
Dr James Warner and Dr Nori Graham
ISBN 978 1 78592 458 3
eISBN 978 1 78450 835 7

Enhancing Health and Wellbeing in Dementia
A Person-Centred Integrated Care Approach
Dr Shibley Rahman
Forewords by Professor Sube Banerjee and Lisa Rodrigues
Afterword by Lucy Frost
ISBN 978 1 78592 037 0
eISBN 978 1 78450 291 1

Supporting People with Dementia in Black, Asian and Minority Ethnic Communities

Key Issues and Strategies for Change

Edited by David Truswell

Foreword by Professor Mark Johnson

Jessica Kingsley *Publishers*
London and Philadelphia

First published in 2020
by Jessica Kingsley Publishers
73 Collier Street
London N1 9BE, UK
and
400 Market Street, Suite 400
Philadelphia, PA 19106, USA

www.jkp.com

Library of Congress Cataloging in Publication Data
A CIP catalog record for this book is available from the Library of Congress

British Library Cataloguing in Publication Data
A CIP catalogue record for this book is available from the British Library

ISBN 978 1 78592 391 3
eISBN 978 1 78450 748 0

Printed and bound in Great Britain

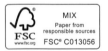

Contents

Foreword

Professor Emeritus Mark R. D. Johnson
UK Centre for Evidence in Ethnicity Health & Diversity
Mary Seacole Research Centre, De Montfort University Leicester

David Truswell and his colleagues are to be congratulated on producing a unique resource – a reader of material relating to dementia among the UK's Black, Asian and minority ethnic (BAME) communities of migrant origin, which combines rigorous academic research, comprehensive reviewing of the relevant literature, and insights based on community views involving both carers and people living with dementia, from a selection of the main groups of the population represented within that broad label. Not before time, they have corrected a historic omission and injustice in the literature on which the design and provision of our health and care services are based. In a sense, this represents a 'coming of age' for the literature on 'ethnic health' – since the times when the predominant issue was the fear of infection from migrants, a fear that remains, however unjustified (Bivins 2015). This was followed by a period where blame was placed on the 'migrants' for failing to understand the national health system or for following 'exotic' cultural behaviours, and a more recent period when attempts were beginning to be made to train healthcare professionals in 'cultural competence'. As the earlier migrants who formed the basis of our post-war (i.e. post-1945) 'minority ethnic' population have aged, and their descendants become the nucleus of a modern British society, new migrants have come to the UK – following in the steps of many earlier generations and cohorts since at least Roman times (Defoe 1701). All of these pose new challenges to the policy makers, practitioners, researchers and trainers of the National Health Service (NHS), which is also waking up itself to the challenge of an ageing 'majority' population and a reported epidemic of dementia across the whole population (All Party Parliamentary Group on Dementia 2014). For once, both majority and minority groups may be facing the challenge together.

The current best estimate is that there are 25,000 people from Black, Asian and minority ethnic backgrounds in England and Wales living with a diagnosis of dementia – a number that is expected to double in the next ten years. However, there is a recognised need to improve rates of early diagnosis and uptake of dementia care services among BAME groups, for whom it is believed there is at present a problem of under-diagnosis, largely because of poor tools and familiarity among practitioners to assess BAME patients. A recent study (Wilson *et al.* 2019) established that GPs may indeed 'estimate' or adjust scores when using the General Practitioner Assessment of Cognition (GPCOG) diagnostic tool 'to take account of language and cultural barriers', so despite a significant number of referrals to memory clinics from these populations (Black and South Asian), many were subsequently diagnosed with other mental health issues. At the same time, referral to the memory clinic was often not valued or desired by families because of a perceived lack of value since there was no 'cure' available, and nor did they expect useful support to be forthcoming. Clearly, GPs respond to the difficulty of diagnosis by referring more BAME people with an 'uncertain' diagnosis, which does not help anyone in the long run. It is to be hoped that the chapters of this book and its clear recommendations may assist in remedying this situation.

The authors open the collection with a quick resumé of the recent past, referencing the work of the All Party Parliamentary Group on Dementia (2013) and Truswell's own review for the Race Equality Foundation (2013). What it does not do, perhaps, is to highlight how this was a well-predicted crisis, foreseen by the charity Age Concern and other researchers in the 1980s (Barker 1984; Ebrahim, Smith and Giggs 1987; Fenton 1987) when considering the UK's lack of experience of dealing with older people from minority ethnic groups, the lack of a resident older cohort of minorities of 'New Commonwealth' origin, and the inevitability of ageing as a group when so many had settled in a short time around the passing of the Commonwealth Immigration Act 1971. That said, it is also too easy to forget that an earlier cohort of Eastern European migrants, especially those of Polish origin, made their homes in Britain following World War II, many as refugees from Nazism and Communism, and they too went through this life-stage – as more recent European migrants will in their turn. These lessons must not be allowed to be forgotten again.

The book continues with a series of 'ethnic-specific' chapters, each of which gives useful background to the migrant origins, history and cultural specificities of the group in question, as well as links to useful resources.

They start with a chapter on the Irish, which usefully underlines that 'minority ethnicity' is not all about skin colour, and it is hoped this will also alert readers to the probability of specific issues arising in other western European origin migrant minority ethnic groups. Tilki also highlights briefly the issue of Gypsy and Irish Travellers in her analysis. A subsequent chapter about the African-Caribbean communities highlights, perhaps unsurprisingly, the issue of racism – which can make the practice of 'reminiscing' therapies problematic – as well as raising the often forgotten notion of an 'African-Caribbean culture'. Too often, being English-speaking people, this has been neglected because of an understanding that sensitivity to culture was synonymous with language and interpreting needs. Not surprisingly, music features here, as with other cultures, as do gender roles and expectations – and maybe we could add 'dominoes' as a pastime?

The chapter on 'Asian' issues is uniquely presented as co-written by a two-generation team of son and mother, both professionals, who succeed in highlighting many learning points as well as the diversity within the Asian communities and the commonalities – most notably the lack of a suitable term for dementia in any major Asian language, and the contrast in attitudes towards 'physical' and mental health conditions. It is also worth underlining the importance of understanding how a collectivist or community-focused worldview differs from the individualist nature of most 'western' societies. One phrase that sticks in my mind: 'Why wouldn't she go back (to her country of birth) in her mind?'

There is much to be learned from two lesser-known or at least more poorly documented groups – the Chinese and the Jewish – as well as some innovative solutions which deserve consideration! It is striking to consider the degree to which both groups have been present over time, and have affected what we consider to be 'our' western culture. The chapters both highlight the degree to which community-based, grassroots organisations have led in innovative service delivery, with lessons that can be transferred not only to other minority groups but also to generic service provision.

Following these 'ethnographic' chapters, a chapter on 'rights' presents a challenging but salutary reminder that there are many issues of inter-sectionality (cross-cutting influences of age, language, disability, culture and discrimination) and legislation which may prove confusing or problematic for carers and others as well as professionals. A useful discussion clearly brings out issues around competence to decide, what the law permits or protects, and how this may affect the professionals' decision making, as anti-discrimination and safeguarding rules interact. There is a selection of case studies and it is important to note that things may not be the same under all legislations – especially in the UK under Scottish law.

Another very valuable section considers in considerable depth the question of spirituality and faith. All too often in a modern, 'rational and scientific' world, too little attention is given to questions of faith, belief and practice of religion, despite the fact that a clear majority of the population in every census or survey admits or claims membership of a faith – those of 'no religion or faith' are a significant but still small minority. And it cannot be denied that patterns of behaviour, values and rituals absorbed in childhood remain and return more strongly in old age. As end of life becomes to be perceived more clearly, what might lie beyond, questions of the intangible and transcendent also gain in salience. Hence, it is essential for the practitioner and service provider to understand more about diversity of faiths, and the support that these and their organisations can offer, in order to best serve the needs of their patients or service users! This might include hymns and sacred songs – such as the 'yoik' communal singing tradition of the Sami people of Scandinavia.

A chapter which many may find hard to read, but which shows considerable courage and reflexivity on the part of its author, is 'a carer's perspective', written by someone who would be seen by most as an expert researcher and academic in the field, who reflects on becoming also an 'expert by experience' and the pain and internal conflict this created. This may also, however, be comforting for those who wonder how they could have not known or noticed things about their own loved ones, and we should be most grateful to Dr Rahman for his honesty as well as the clear and insightful academic discussion he provides.

The book concludes with a summary which speaks for itself, highlighting the centrality of identity – a key leitmotiv of the 21st century – showing how this is intimately tied up with 'race', culture and faith, and the experience of being (or becoming) 'other' in an often-hostile society. It makes clear and vital recommendations, such as reference to the need for a national Resource Hub, training and funding, including attention to the issue of additional costs, and calling for an inclusive future strategy. Finally, there is an excellent set of links to further useful resources. For this alone, the book will become a useful reference on anyone's bookshelf!

References

All Party Parliamentary Group on Dementia (2013) *Dementia does not discriminate: The experiences of black, Asian and minority ethnic communities*. London: All Party Parliamentary Group on Dementia.

All Party Parliamentary Group on Dementia (2014) *Building on the National Dementia Strategy: Change, progress and priorities*. London: All Party Parliamentary Group on Dementia.

Barker, J. (1984) *Black and Asian Old People in Britain*. Mitcham: Age Concern.

Bivins, R. (2015) *Contagious Communities: Medicine, Migration, and the NHS in Post War Britain*. Oxford: Oxford University Press.

Defoe, D. (1701) 'The True Born Englishman.' Reprinted (1995) *British Medical Journal* 313, 145.

Ebrahim, S., Smith, C. and Giggs, J. (1987) 'Elderly Immigrants – a disadvantaged group?' *Age and Ageing*, 16, 4, 249–255.

Fenton, S. (1987) *Ageing Minorities: Black People as they Grow Old in Britain*. London: Commission for Racial Equality.

Truswell D. (2013) *Black and minority ethnic communities and dementia: Where are we now?* Race Equality Foundation Briefing Paper.

Wilson, A., Subramanian, H., Raghavan, R., Johnson M.R.D., *et al.* (2019) 'Diagnosis and management of dementia in primary care in Black Asian and Minority Ethnic groups: an exploratory study.' *Final Report to National Institute of Health Research* (PB-PG-0416-200019).

Note on Terminology and Diagnosis

Throughout this book, the authors will use the term dementia in a general way that refers to Alzheimer's disease, the most common form of dementia, and vascular dementia, a form of dementia more usually associated with the outcome of stroke and the second most common form of dementia. Mainstream media reports and UK policy documents usually use the term dementia in this way. Dementia is a group of related symptoms that arise out of diseases that affect the brain. The most common one is Alzheimer's disease, affecting 1 in 14 people over the age of 65 in the UK. About 60 per cent of people living with dementia have Alzheimer's disease and about 20 per cent of those living with dementia have vascular dementia (Rizzi, Rosset and Roriz-Cruz, 2014).

The Alzheimer's Society website[1] is a good general online resource for more information about these and other types of dementia.

While loss of short-term memory can be one of the early signs of dementia, the gradual pervasive damage to the brain caused by the illness can manifest in many other ways, as the various testimonies of individual experience in this book demonstrate. Other health problems apart from dementia can lead to memory problems, and dementia can affect those under 65. Anyone with worries about persisting health problems that affect concentration, memory, intellectual functioning or mood should seek advice from their GP. Problems with tasks that involve thinking, calculating, recognising or doing things in a familiar sequence may often be part of the early signs. There may be changes in mood or temperament. As the illness progresses, these changes will become more frequent and persist for longer. An important emphasis in this book is to encourage people from Black, Asian and minority ethnic (BAME) communities, especially older people, who are worried about their health to seek GP advice rather than dismiss and minimise the problems as 'just part of getting old'.

Reference

Rizzi, L., Rosset, I. and Roriz-Cruz, M. (2014) 'Global epidemiology of dementia: Alzheimer's and vascular types.' *BioMed Research International* 2014:908915.

---

1   www.alzheimers.org.uk

CHAPTER 1

Introduction

David Truswell

The 2013 report *Dementia does not discriminate* by the All Party Parliamentary Group on Dementia was an important milestone in the recognition of the impact of dementia on UK Black, Asian and minority ethnic (BAME) communities, looking at both the status of research on dementia in BAME communities at the time and taking in a broad range of testimony on the experience of individuals and organisations. At around the same time, I completed a briefing paper for the Race Equality Foundation (Truswell 2013) that reviewed UK research literature over the previous five years and looked at several examples of grassroots organisations taking action to raise awareness about dementia in BAME communities and provide information and support to the communities. The work was supported by the Central and North West London (CNWL) NHS Foundation Trust as part of a project looking at raising awareness about dementia in BAME communities to improve take-up of the organisation's memory services. This work also later produced an internal guidance document for CNWL's memory services (Truswell and Tavera 2016).

The subsequent years have seen a slowly rising awareness across the health and social care mainstream of the need to recognise that there are issues specific to the experience of BAME communities that introduce a further layer of complexity to the already complex and life-changing challenges facing those living with dementia, and their families and carers. However, the individual research papers and articles remain scarce and often reflect pilot-level studies that are limited to a few dozen research participants. With the notable exception in the UK of Julia Botsford's and Karen Harrison Dening's (2015) *Dementia, Culture and Ethnicity*, there is a dearth of texts that attempt to capture the full range of issues that affect those from BAME communities living with dementia, and their families and carers.

I am indebted to a number of people with an in-depth experience of the impact of dementia who have collaborated with me to produce this book, either by writing individual chapters, writing chapters in collaboration with me or contributing material from their own experiences. The contributors cover a wide range of backgrounds and a number speak from personal experience of living with dementia or supporting family members living with dementia as well as those sharing their professional knowledge and experience. An important aim of this book is to show the many perspectives there are to the story of BAME communities living with dementia, underpinning this with accounts of personal experience and making reference to the available research evidence. The book will be of interest to professionals working with people from BAME communities, those from BAME communities who would like to know more about how dementia is affecting their communities, those who are living with dementia from BAME communities and those who are their carers. These last two groups of people often find themselves desperately looking for any information on dementia that reflects some of the experience of BAME communities.

Individual chapters in the book stand alone with the intention of allowing the reader to dip in and out of the book as a reference resource. Initially, the chapters on specific communities focus on some of the most long-standing UK BAME communities with demographically high proportions of people who are over 65. Subsequent chapters deal with the issues that have a commonality across BAME communities. This includes a detailed account of the experience of one BAME carer, Dr Shibley Rahman, which encapsulates a number of the issues mentioned by the previous authors as well as elaborating on the experience of the often-neglected issue of delirium in dementia.

Although there are many BAME communities that have made their home in the UK over the generations, much more work remains to be done to examine and understand the impact of dementia on the full range of these communities. While BAME communities collectively have a demographic profile that is younger than the mainstream White UK community, a more finely grained understanding of the migration history of UK BAME communities shows a variety of age demographics across ethnic communities. This reflects their different histories of settlement, for example post-World War II or even earlier migration, refugees from late 20th- and early 21st-century conflicts or political upheavals, and migration in the more recent period of European Union (EU) integration and enlargement. However, there are valuable lessons to be learned in looking at the commonalties across those migrant populations with an older demographic profile that will reduce the likelihood of needing to 'reinvent the wheel' as newer and younger migrant populations age and decide to stay in the UK. The challenges dementia creates for migrant communities and the services that support migrant communities living with dementia are worldwide (Truswell 2016).

I was fortunate in having Dr Mary Tilki and Dr Karan Jutlla, with her mother Harjinder Kaur co-authoring, writing about the Irish and South Asian communities, respectively. These authors have written extensively about these communities over the years and are rightly respected for their perspective and contribution to the research evidence and depth of personal knowledge of the communities they write about. Formal research into the impact of dementia in the African-Caribbean community is limited and I am indebted to individuals who have contributed their personal stories to help bring to light the experience of people from this community and to Culture Dementia UK for the many opportunities it has provided to hear from and speak to people in the African-Caribbean community living with dementia or supporting those living with dementia. Padraic Garrett's chapter on the Jewish community, and the support provided by Tom Lam and Gill Tam to produce the chapter on the Chinese community, have provided comprehensive accounts of two communities that are rarely considered in UK dementia research literature yet have a long and rich cultural and economic historical relationship within the UK and significant numbers of older members living in the UK. Importantly, organisations such as Jewish Care and the Chinese National Healthy Living Centre have done significant work with their respective communities at a scale that would warrant examination and investment by mainstream dementia service commissioners, not simply to improve services for these communities but for examples of freshness, creativity and direct involvement with the whole community in awareness-raising that the mainstream could learn much from.

In looking at common issues, I was fortunate to have the assistance of people who have been working and writing for some time on the areas focused on for this book. Toby Williamson, a writer and researcher on a rights-based approach in dementia, brings his knowledge and experience to a detailed examination of how the different levels of understanding of 'rights' come into play for those in BAME communities living with dementia, and their families and carers. Setting this in the context of case examples, he brings into focus how the complex balance of interests and rights can play out in individual situations, moving the conversation about living with dementia on from a narrow focus on health and care needs to a wider examination of quality of life.

Dr Natalie Tolbert has written extensively on spirituality and mental health, the limitations of western models of medicine and the role of personal faith in healing, including its role in mental health. In Chapter 8 we critically explore the recent research on the role of faith and spirituality in dementia and look at how both personal faith and community beliefs can either be a barrier to living well with dementia or a source of support and benefit. We also consider how personal spirituality is not confined to those with a professed religion.

In an overarching chapter (Chapter 9), I cover briefly several themes that often arise in practice or in conversations with people from BAME communities but are rarely a focus in the research literature: interpreting and translation, supplementary costs of care for BAME communities, the lack of appropriate reminiscence materials, and end-of life care. One general problem not mentioned in this chapter is the cultural limitation of diagnostic tools for memory assessment, as this is referred to in some detail in a number of the personal accounts and also within the chapters focused on the experience of different communities.

I am deeply indebted to Dr Shibley Rahman for his account of his personal experience as a son coming to terms with becoming a 'partner in care' for his mother as they both come to terms with her living with dementia. This sets the context for the BAME carer in Chapter 10 on one person's experience of being a carer. Also, his chapter deals with the experience of living with delirium in dementia, an issue rarely spoken of in the research literature from the perspective of the carer.

Just as dementia itself is not just one thing, the additional challenge dementia brings to people from BAME communities is not just one thing. This book brings together a set of perspectives or vantage points with varying significance for people as a result of their own experience of living with dementia. The different authors throughout the book point to issues that are likely to be of importance to people from BAME backgrounds living with dementia or helpful in supporting them or their families. The significance of particular aspects of culture will vary over the course of the illness and between individuals.

When exploring the cultural issues for BAME people living with dementia, and their family and carers, we are looking at the personal experience and meaning for the individual, what matters to them and where their sense of support comes from, rather than trying to figure out or tell anyone which culture box they need to tick. Dr Rahman's chapter is eloquent in illustrating this as he recounts how he and his mother have moved to talking Bangladeshi now and how his relationship has in some ways changed in becoming a carer but in some ways hasn't because he's doing what a son should do. The shifts and realignments of roles and feelings about roles (e.g. father/daughter, husband/wife, grandmother/grandchild) are echoed in a number of other personal accounts throughout the book. These shifts are filtered through ideas and convictions about 'face', faith, filial obligation, duty and love in many different ways. The different ways this happens for individuals is also a glimpse of how cultural differences are expressed within people's daily lives as they live with dementia. Linda, a carer who reccounts her experience in the book, refers to this as 'learning to parent the parent'.

The concluding chapter summarises the wide-ranging contributions and introduces a set of ambitious proposals intended to give a broader direction to information and service developments in the UK, which currently rely too much on local but largely isolated champions, whether they be within or external to the local health and care institutional arrangements. There does need to be a significant step-up in scale from local pilots involving relatively small numbers of participants to more substantial and more widely beneficial systemic change. This is vital if we are to make an impact on the scale of the challenge posed by the increase dementia rate in BAME communities identified in 2013 by the All-Party Parliamentary Group on Dementia. This step-up currently is nowhere in sight.

References

All Party Parliamentary Group on Dementia (2013) *Dementia does not discriminate: The experiences of black, Asian and minority ethnic communities.* London: All Party Parliamentary Group on Dementia.

Botsford, J. and Harrison Denning, K. (2015) *Dementia, Culture and Ethnicity: Issues for All.* London: Jessica Kingsley Publishers.

Truswell, D. (2013) *Black, Asian and Minority Ethnic Communities and Dementia – Where Are We Now?* Better Health Briefing Paper 30. London: Race Equality Foundation. Available at: https://raceequalityfoundation.org.uk/wp-content/uploads/2018/03/health-30.pdf.

Truswell, D. (2016) 'The impact of dementia on migrant communities: A complex challenge in a globalised world.' *Alzheimer's, Dementia and Cognitive Neurology* 1. doi: 10.15761/ADCN.1000102.

Truswell, D. and Tavera, Y. (2016) *An Electronic Resource Handbook for CNWL Memory Services: Dementia Information for Black, Asian and Minority Ethnic Communities.* London: Central and North West London NHS Foundation Trust. Available at: www. cnwl.nhs.uk/wp-content/uploads/Memory-Services-Handbook-final.pdf.

CHAPTER 2

Dementia and Irish People in Britain

Dr Mary Tilki

The reader might be surprised to find a chapter about Irish people in a text relating to dementia among Black, Asian and minority ethnic (BAME) or migrant communities. This is because migration, ethnicity and inequality debates in the UK have largely neglected the Irish community in Britain (Tilki 2015). Defining ethnicity in a Black/White skin colour paradigm has the effect of making the White (mostly) English-speaking Irish invisible. Although data on Irish ethnicity and place of birth is collected, it is mainly presented within the overall White category, thus presuming the Irish are the same as the majority and other White populations. More importantly, it neglects the health and social inequalities which Irish people in Britain have experienced for decades (Tilki 2003, 2015; Tilki *et al.* 2009). The Irish are not a homogeneous group and although many have been successful in Britain, the profile of the majority is more akin to that of other BAME groups than the majority population.

The 2011 census shows a distinctive age profile for the Irish community in Britain, with a higher proportion of people above 55 and particularly beyond pension age than in the general or minority ethnic populations (Ryan *et al.* 2014). This reflects migration patterns, with 38 per cent of the Irish community arriving before 1961 and a further 18 per cent between 1961 and 1971 (Ryan *et al.* 2014). Although Irish people have high levels of employment, especially in upper occupational categories, a large proportion of the community is economically inactive due to retirement (Ryan *et al.* 2014). In addition, significant numbers from about 50 upwards and Irish Travellers of working age are economically inactive because of long-term sickness or disability (Ryan *et al.* 2014). Reflecting the demographic profile of the community, Irish people are more likely to be living in single-person households than any other group in England, with consequent implications for care and support in old age and illness (Tilki *et al.* 2009). While age is probably the most significant risk for dementia among the Irish community, this is magnified by the poor health and social isolation they experience. Truswell (2013) estimates that there are around 10,000 Irish people in England with dementia.

The 2011 census provides robust evidence of high levels of limiting long-term illness (LLTI) and self-reported poor health among Irish people over 50 (Ryan *et al.* 2014). Gypsy and Irish Travellers aged 50 and over have the highest levels of LLTI and 'bad' or 'very bad' health in England. Research by Irish community organisations suggests that mobility problems, cardiovascular disease, pain, cancer, depression and anxiety are common causes of LLTI (Moore *et al.* 2012). Research demonstrates that Irish people have disproportionately high rates of heart disease, hypertension and stroke, particularly in older age bands (British Heart Foundation 2010; Harding, Rosato and Teyhan 2008; Wild *et al.* 2007). The incidence of mental illness among Irish communities is high, with high levels of common mental disorders (Weich *et al.* 2004), excessive rates of depression, anxiety and psychological ill-health (Ryan *et al.* 2006) and high admission rates especially at older ages (Care Quality Commission and National Mental Health Development Unit 2010). Given the poor health profile, it is not surprising that a quarter of Irish people and over 40 per cent of Gypsy and Irish Travellers provide 50 or more hours of unpaid care each week (Ryan *et al.* 2014). These factors increase the risk of social isolation.

Like other minority ethnic groups, Irish people moved to Britain to escape poverty, find work and better themselves. They rarely expected to settle, intending to return in four or five years having gained a qualification or saved a particular amount of money (Tilki 2003). Most left their home country for economic reasons, pulled by and directly recruited to jobs in particular sectors of the labour market. They often left to join siblings or to get away from claustrophobic towns and villages already depopulated of young people.

The author acknowledges the commonalities experienced by all people with dementia and their carers, but this chapter emphasises some of the differences which might not be appreciated in health and social care settings. As recent memory becomes difficult to access, people with dementia rely on memories from earlier periods in their lives. These can be comforting but also can be vivid and distressing and often manifest as unusual behaviour. Understanding the biography and experiences of a person living with dementia underpins and facilitates person-centred, culturally sensitive care. This chapter will outline the experience of older Irish migrants, highlighting the difficulties many encountered, which shaped their attitude to British society and health services.

It will also explore differences in culture and language which differentiate them from the majority population and how these become more relevant when people have dementia. The discussion will be illustrated with quotes from the author's research, community consultations and life stories from Irish third-sector organisations.

Similarities but differences

It might be very easy to assume that the Irish are the same as the English, given that they look similar and speak the same language. While there are shared experiences, having spent a lifetime in the same locality, there are also many differences. These become more important when people develop dementia, when recent memories fail and those of earlier times become more accessible.

While Irish people may have lived and worked in the same neighbourhood for decades, it is a mistake to assume that they will all feel comfortable with mainstream services in their area. Many feel they have never fitted in because of experiences when they first migrated and at different times since (Tilki 2017). The feelings that shaped their memories may become more vivid when recent memory is fragile. Most Irish people found the English polite, but they still felt like outsiders rather than part of the workplace or community. Although Irish people worked in farms, factories and hospitals alongside the English during World War II, they were seen as a threat to national security and persistently taunted about Ireland's neutrality (Tilki *et al.* 2010). While the English appeared formal, when Irish people tried to find somewhere to live, they faced hostility.

> When I came to England there was no blacks, no dogs, no Irish. I remember seeing an ad for a flat in the post office. She banged the door in our faces when she heard the accent. Bloody Irish! Slam! (Kay)

From the late 1960s, 'The Troubles' in Northern Ireland legitimated public expressions of anti-Irish racism and draconian police powers through the Prevention of Terrorism Act (PTA) 1974. Every Irish person was suspected of allegiance to the Irish Republican Army and, as such, complicit in terrorism.

> I remember being in the gardens at the back of my house the time of the Hyde Park bombing. I had my five children with me. I was ordered out of the gardens. I knew nothing about it. (Margaret)

I had it with patients. I remember going on to the orthopaedic ward; 'The Irish and the bombs. Ye're all the same'. (Philomena, staff nurse)

Survival for Irish people meant keeping a low profile, avoiding speaking, or trying to conceal their accent. Irishness was only expressed in the privacy of home, Catholic Church, dancing school or local Irish centre. Those difficult times generated discomfort and guardedness among the older generation.

While Irish people do not have the same language problems as other minorities, communication can still be problematic. Although English speaking, they speak with different accents, expressions or terms for common items, often reflecting translation from the Irish language. Irish family names and first names can be difficult to pronounce and it can add to the confusion of a person with dementia when their name is mispronounced. The mother tongue of a small number of people from Gaeltacht (Irish-speaking) areas is Irish, with English learned as a second language on migration. The ability to communicate in the second language can be lost when the person has dementia.

Older Irish people are especially sensitive about having to repeat themselves or having their accents mimicked in public and professional settings.

With the English doctors, you have to keep repeating yourself – it's embarrassing. When you say something the way we do, they correct you and make you feel very, very little. Or they take the mickey out of your accent. (Alice)

Sadly, the feeling of not being safe outside family and community was further perpetuated by Irish people's experiences of health professionals. Older people repeatedly recounted consultations where the first question the doctor asked was about alcohol consumption (Tilki 2003). Furthermore, they were not believed if they said they were abstainers or only had an occasional drink

One of the first questions the doctor is likely to ask is 'Do you drink?' and if you admit to taking a drop at all, it's automatically assumed that you are an alcoholic and that's the cause of all your problems. (Michael)

I said to him 'Doctor, I don't drink,' and he said 'What? An Irish person who doesn't drink?' I was furious. (Bridget)

Overt and insinuated anti-Irish racism instilled insecurity, a lack of confidence and a strategy of keeping heads down. Today, this may explain the reticence of older Irish people in non-Irish settings. Although people have dealt with their insecurities over the years, reliving painful emotions when memory fails can recreate the anxieties of the past. This may contribute to agitation, unusual behaviour or negative responses to doctors or other professionals by Irish people with dementia.

Cultural sensitivity for older Irish people

It is important that services for people with dementia are welcoming and navigable. For the reasons mentioned in the previous section, Irish people are likely to be reluctant to access services for mainstream elders or dementia. This is exacerbated by practical issues such as poor health, poverty and lack of transport, which prevent people participating in activities outside the home. Although Irish people are reluctant to use mainstream services, they are often unwilling to use Irish services unless recommended by a trusted person. Therefore, many Irish organisations provide outreach to older, isolated or marginalised people using culturally sensitive staff or volunteers.

There is undeniable stigma around dementia, so Irish organisations focus on being welcoming and non-judgemental. They value confidentiality while encouraging people to be open, talk about difficulties in a safe environment, share experiences and help them recognise the structural roots of problems, rather than blaming themselves. In particular, they operate a strengths model, recognising problems, but focusing on and capturing the strengths and resilience of the individuals involved.

Elders services are increasingly adopting Dementia Engagement and Empowerment Project (DEEP) guidance for dementia-inclusive environments,[1] but it is also important to take account of culture for people from minority ethnic groups. Traditional images of shamrocks, harps and leprechauns may seem old-fashioned but can be very meaningful and comforting to vulnerable Irish people or those with dementia. Posters, photographs, county coats of arms, Irish background music and familiar accents help people feel safe and at home.

---

1 www.dementiavoices.org.uk/deep-guides/for-organisations-and-communities

I enjoyed the local clubs, but Paddy was restless, withdrawn and unhappy. The only place he relaxed was at the Irish lunch club. He could have a laugh and a joke... As his condition deteriorated and his speech was muddled, his face would light up when he heard the accents. He was with his own people. (Rita, carer, London)

Stimulation and social interaction for Irish people with dementia are facilitated through conversation, exercise, bingo, card games and culturally appropriate memory work.

I look forward to coming and recounting old times with the others. I enjoy the memory sessions each Thursday, meeting with friends all suffering from memory loss. (Michael, service user with dementia, Leeds)

Irish music is a major focus of activities in Irish community organisations for all participants, and plays a key role in expressing emotions by people with dementia (Tilki *et al.* 2010). Memory for familiar music is particularly well preserved, even in people with advanced stages of dementia (Vella-Burrows 2012), and can enhance recall of personal memories (El Haj, Postal and Allain 2012). Background music can calm agitation and aggression and increase sensory awareness and communication (Garabedian 2014). Music can be recorded or live, but singing is particularly valuable in dementia (Wall and Duffy 2010). Singing helps with language, and people with dementia find great joy in interacting with others and remembering the songs they sang as children.

Research evidence about the value of physical activity in dementia is controversial (Guure *et al.* 2017; Sabia *et al.* 2017). However, it is clear that exercise improves wellbeing and offers enjoyment. Irish organisations provide exercise sessions for people of differing physical abilities. 'Tea Dances' are highly popular afternoon events, offering social interaction, exercise and continuity as people maintain the traditions of their youth and recall the Irish dance halls they frequented as young people. While some may be too frail to engage in physically demanding 'sets' or 'céilís', many are able to enjoy a gentle waltz. This provides physical exercise but also affords opportunities for reminiscence and social interaction and may be the only physical contact an isolated person has all week.

Irish organisations invariably provide Irish newspapers, films and DVDs and variously incorporate them into discussions which stimulate verbal abilities, promote conversation and enable people to keep up to date with current events. Requiem masses, wakes, funerals and memorial services are an important part of Irish culture, demonstrating respect for and celebrating the lives of deceased members of the community. Rather than being morbid or reminding people of their own immortality, they are often reassuring and comforting, especially for those without family (Tilki *et al.* 2010).

Reminiscence

Reminiscence is a popular activity among services for people with dementia. It relies on sharing life experiences, memories and stories from the past. It is an enjoyable activity, which captures the ability of people to recall the past when recent memories are less accessible. It is said to improve quality of life, reduce agitation and offer a sense of competence and confidence as people use their retained skills to recall past events (Woods *et al.* 2012). It also provides an opening for people to get to know each other through shared experiences and can allow staff to get to know 'the person' with dementia rather than a person with dementia. This can facilitate an individualised plan of care as well as a better understanding of behaviour.

> During a Happy Days reminiscence session, we were talking about what it was like going to school in Ireland and how it differs from today. The participants recalled how the children would write on a slate with chalk. A slate was passed around the group so they could all use the chalk.
>
> One woman with advanced dementia needed a lot of encouragement to take part. As the slate got to her she started to write with the chalk. We didn't recognise what she had written, but when asked she said it was her name in Irish. Her daughter was shocked as she didn't know that her mother had learnt Irish or could write her name in Irish. This was an emotional moment for her daughter. She got her mother to write her name on paper, which the daughter keeps as a lovely memory. (Irish Community Services, Greenwich, Bexley and Lewisham)

Had the group in this situation not been culturally sensitive, the importance of what the woman had written might have been dismissed as meaningless, rather than providing opportunities for her family or the Happy Days group to encourage her to take part.

Reminiscence can also retrieve bad memories. It should be undertaken by staff who are culturally competent and who have facilitation skills. In the Irish context, this means understanding the Irish migratory experience, anticipating and being sensitive to grief, pain and loss which may have been buried for decades. Facilitators should be adept in handling sadness at leaving home, bereavement, discrimination in Ireland and Britain, perceptions of failure, not being able to return home and ending their days in another country (Tilki *et al.* 2010).

Understanding behaviour

Recent advances in dementia research suggest that behaviour which might be considered 'challenging' is not meaningless but a way of communicating distress or suffering or a response to the social and physical environment. Most changes in behaviour come from heightened levels of stress which can be caused by physical, psychological, environmental or communication factors. Pain, hunger, anxiety, embarrassment, and inability to navigate the environment or express themselves are very common causes of distress. Unless the underlying cause of the behaviour or the function it serves are understood, it can be difficult to alleviate (Krishnamoorthy and Anderson 2011). For example, repeatedly not being understood can make a person angry or withdrawn, in danger of being labelled difficult or less competent than they really are.

Clearly, every person with dementia is different and the way in which the condition manifests is individual. Knowing the person with dementia as a person can not only help explain why somebody comes across as difficult, but facilitate strategies to make the person more secure and comfortable. The preceding sections highlight some of the memories which might make an Irish person with dementia anxious, unsure or reluctant to engage with. Those harassed or arrested under the PTA may react aggressively to being touched, taken to the bathroom or seeing somebody with a dark uniform or a tone of voice that reminds them of a police officer. Irish Travellers are particularly sensitive, having experienced forced evictions by the police and hostility from the public. Remembering such experiences may explain anger and verbal or physical aggression, for example when helping to mobilise or bathe somebody or move them by ambulance.

Even earlier memories can trigger negative responses. Apart from economic reasons, many Irish people left Ireland to get away from an unfair, religiously authoritarian society. Abuses experienced in institutions or the family may emerge in reminiscence or when the person is freed from inhibitions which kept such matters 'secret'. Irish child-rearing practices were often harsh and some people will have lived in abusive families. However, a significant number of young Irish people left Ireland in the 1950s and 1960s to escape abuse in religious institutions.

> I was in an orphanage you know. Physically, emotionally, sexually abused – terrible, terrible. I was 16 when I came here. As soon I got out I came over here [to England]. (Martin)

Some have had help to address these traumas but many have repressed them and kept them hidden throughout their lives. Feeling cold or hungry, being left in the dark, touched by somebody unfamiliar or undressed for bathing can trigger traumatic memories, which may manifest as crying, swearing or physical aggression.

The nature of Irish society also meant that many pregnant unmarried girls and gay people of both sexes fled to the anonymity of England, carrying these 'secrets' often for the rest of their lives. Some may never have told their families, or families who did know might fear that dementia could lead to disclosure. These 'secrets' have implications for staff and volunteers and must be handled sensitively, ethically and, if necessary, by appropriate professionals.

Services for carers, respite and advocacy

Like other BAME groups, there is a high level of informal care within the Irish community, with a significant proportion of carers providing 50 or more hours' care per week especially among Irish Travellers (Ryan *et al.* 2014; Tilki 2015; Tilki *et al.* 2009). Many do not consider themselves carers and see this as part of their role as wives, husbands or daughters (Tilki *et al.* 2009). As in wider society, carers are often old, frail and in deteriorating health. Most have little knowledge about what is available, but many Irish people fear that if they ask for help, the person they care for will be placed in residential care.

In addition to lunch clubs, memory groups or dementia cafes which offer a brief respite for carers, some Irish organisations provide specific facilities for carers. Increasingly, organisations facilitate carers' support groups, which encourage carers to socialise, share problems and support each other. Advice is offered about coping with the person with dementia, avoiding back and other injuries and handling the abuse that carers often experience. One innovative initiative is a sitting-in service for carers where trained Disclosure and Barring Service (DBS)-checked volunteers sit with the person with dementia while the carer has a break for a few hours.

Much of the work of Irish organisations in Britain is providing information about benefits and services and especially about dementia diagnosis, treatment and management. Advice workers assist families in applying for allowances or, more commonly, appealing decisions about benefits or care services. Organisations provide advocacy around the same problems that other carers experience, such as care services, home adaptations, respite care or related matters. However, Irish families frequently have an additional barrier to overcome – recognition of the cultural needs of the Irish person with dementia. While acknowledging that the cultural needs of BAME people are far from perfect, it is commonly assumed that services for the majority population suit the Irish. Casework from community organisations report that Irish families who ask whether it is possible to have an Irish careworker are frequently told they cannot make such requests. Those who have asked have been perceived to be racist (Tilki *et al.* 2010).

Why Irish community organisations?

Although mainstream services are well intentioned, they are often inadvertently ethnocentric. The following story from an Irish community organisation not only highlights the importance of accent but how a knowledge of the person could have shaped some of the activities which might have relieved some of her unhappiness.

I was approached by a care home to make contact with Mrs M from Wicklow who was living with dementia. On my first visit, I found her to be very isolated and depressed, and heavily medicated. I introduced myself and she immediately remembered my family, my Irish connections and began to reminiscence. She told me that staff and residents in the care home were unable to understand her accent. They thought she was less able mentally than she actually was, which she found frustrating. They thought she was awkward and avoided her as much as possible.

As I got to know her, she told me that her son had passed away and her daughter rarely visited, so she had nobody to talk to. We talked about her life in Ireland, the death of her mother when she was a child, being unable to marry the person she loved as her father did not approve, coming to England and marrying somebody abusive. Her childhood memories were different from most of the other residents. Activities, songs, local history and stories were based around Lancashire childhoods, so meant little to Mrs M. Mrs M died soon afterwards, but the care home did not let me know so I was unable to attend her funeral or pay my respects, which is an important part of Irish culture. (Maxine, Irish Community Care, Liverpool)

The Cuimhne Project – a whole-community response to dementia

'Cuimhne' pronounced 'queevna' is the Irish word for memory, and the Cuimhne Irish Memory Loss Alliance is a whole-community response to dementia in the Irish community in Britain. Mapping and consultation with Irish organisations in Britain in 2010 identified that the numbers of people with suspected or confirmed dementia using services for elders had been increasing for several years (Federation of Irish Societies 2010). They were especially concerned that people with dementia and their carers were dropping out of lunch clubs and social events. Advice and advocacy services were inundated with requests to help families negotiate the health and care system, which was rarely accessed until a crisis happened. Organisations were confident to provide culturally sensitive services for older people but did not necessarily feel equipped to provide the correct support for people living with dementia.

The Cuimhne Project was established in 2013 to raise awareness of dementia in the Irish community and to build an alliance of community organisations, businesses, religious, sport and cultural groups to support and extend knowledge and endeavour to reduce stigma. It also aimed to develop and strengthen support networks through partnerships with mainstream and third-sector bodies, sharing knowledge, and learning from each other. Considerable effort went into representation, reminding relevant parts of national and local government and major charities of their responsibility to address the neglect of health and social care inequalities experienced by Irish taxpayers living with dementia. Over the first four years of Cuimhne, almost 300 volunteers and a smaller number of staff in over 20 Irish organisations across England received dementia awareness training. Community organisations felt encouraged to provide more focused services such as dementia cafes, reminiscence sessions, carers support, music and oral history activities. This work is predominantly funded by the Emigrant Support Project of the Irish government, generous sponsorship and donations and some funding for London from the City Bridge Trust. Irish businesses have contributed in cash and kind and continue to support local community projects. This is only the tip of the iceberg but the principles of the Cuimhne Project are adaptable and applicable beyond the Irish community.

References

British Heart Foundation (2010) *Ethnic Differences on Cardiovascular Disease*. London: British Heart Foundation.

Care Quality Commission and National Mental Health Development Unit (2010) *Count Me In 2010 – The National Mental Health and Learning Disability Census*. London: Care Quality Commission and National Mental Health Development Unit.

El Haj, M., Postal, V. and Allain, P. (2012) 'Music enhances autobiographical memory in mild Alzheimers disease.' *Educational Gerontology*, 38, 1, 30–41. Available at: www.tandfonline.com/doi/abs/10.1080/03601277.2010.515897.

Federation of Irish Societies (2010) *Mapping Services for Elders within the Irish Community A factsheet analysing elders' services, with particular focus on lunch club provision and dementia services*. London: Federation of Irish Societies.

Garabedian, C. (2014) 'I'd Rather Have Music!': The Effects of Live and Recorded Music for People with Dementia Living in Care Homes, and their Carers. PhD thesis. Available at: https://dspace.stir.ac.uk/bitstream/1893/21757/3/POSTVIVA%20THESIS%2013%20FINAL%20May%202015.pdf.

Guure, C., Ibrahim, N., Adam, M. and Said, S. (2017) 'Impact of physical activity on cognitive decline, dementia, and its subtypes: meta-analysis of prospective studies.' *Biomed Research International*. Available at: www.hindawi.com/journals/bmri/2017/9016924.

Harding, S., Rosato, M. and Teyhan, A. (2008) 'Trends for coronary health disease and stroke mortality among migrants in England and Wales: Slow declines for some groups.' *Heart*, 94, 463–470.

Krishnamoorthy, A. and Anderson, D. (2011) 'Managing challenging behaviour in older adults with dementia.' Available at: https://doi.org/10.1002/pnp.199.

Moore, J., Waters, E., Tilki, M. and Clarke, L. (2012) *Fresh Perspectives: A Needs Analysis of the Irish Community in London*. London: London Irish Centre/Federation of Irish Societies.

Ryan, L., Leavey, G., Golden, A., Blizard, R. and King, M. (2006) 'Depression in Irish migrants living in London. A case control study.' *British Journal of Psychiatry*, 188: 560–566.

Ryan, L., D'Angelo, A., Puniskis, M. and Kaye, N. (2014) *Analysis of 2011 Census Data. Irish Community Statistics, England and Selected Urban Areas.* Irish in Britain, Middlesex University. Available at: www.irishinbritain.org/cmsfiles/Downloads/Reports/Irish-Census-Analysis-Report---London.pdf.

Sabia, S., Dugravot, A., Dartigues, J.F., Abell, J. *et al.* (2017) 'Physical activity, cognitive decline, and risk of dementia: 28 year follow-up of Whitehall II cohort study.' *British Medical Journal.* Available at: www.bmj.com/content/357/bmj.j2709.

Tilki, M. (2003) 'A Study of the Health of Irish Born People in London: The Relevance of Social and Economic Factors, Health Beliefs and Behaviour.' Unpublished PhD thesis. London: Middlesex University. Available at: http://eprints.mdx.ac.uk/6724.

Tilki, M. (2015) *Dementia and Cancer in the Irish Community in Britain.* Better Health Briefing Paper 38. London: Race Equality Foundation. Available at: www. irishinbritain.org/cmsfiles/Better-Health-Briefing---Dementia-and-Cancer-in-the-Irish-Community-2.pdf.

Tilki, M. (2017) 'Forgotten but not gone: Older Irish with dementia in England.' *Journal of Dementia Care* 5, (3), 30–31.

Tilki, M., Mulligan, E., Pratt, E., Halley, E. and Taylor, E. (2010) 'Older Irish people with dementia in England.' *Advances in Mental Health*, 9, 3, 21–23.

Tilki, M., Ryan, L., D'Angelo, A. and Sales, R. (2009) *The Forgotten Irish.* Report of a research project commissioned by Ireland Fund of Great Britain. London: Ireland Fund of Great Britain. Available at: http://eprints.mdx.ac.uk/6350/1/Tilki-Forgotten_Irish.pdf.

Truswell, D. (2013) *Black, Asian and Minority Ethnic Communities and Dementia – Where Are We Now?* Better Health Briefing Paper 30. London: Race Equality Foundation. Available at: https://raceequalityfoundation.org.uk/wp-content/uploads/2018/03/health-30.pdf.

Vella-Burrows, T. (2012) *Singing and People with Dementia.* Folkstone: Sidney de Haan Research Centre for Arts and Health/Canterbury Christchurch University. Available at: www.canterbury.ac.uk/health-and-wellbeing/sidney-de-haan-research-centre/documents/singing-and-people-with-dementia.pdf.

Wall, M. and Duffy, A. (2010) 'The effects of music therapy for older people with dementia.' *British Journal of Nursing*, 19, 2, 108–113. Available at: www.ncbi.nlm.nih.gov/pubmed/20220649.

Wild, S., Fischbacher, C., Brick, A., Griffiths C. and Bhopla, R. (2007) 'Mortality for all causes and circulatory disease by country of birth in England and Wales 2001–2003.' *Journal of Public Health*, 29, 2, 191–198.

Weich, S., Nazroo, J., Sproston, K. *et al.* (2004) 'Common mental disorders and ethnicity in England. The EMPIRIC study.' *Psychological Medicine*, 34, 1543–1551.

Woods, R., Bruce, E., Edwards, R.T., Elvish, R. *et al.* (2012) 'REMCARE: reminiscence groups for people with dementia and their family caregivers – effectiveness and cost-effectiveness pragmatic multicentre randomised trial.' *Health Technology Assessment*, 16, (48). Available at: www.ncbi.nlm.nih.gov/books/NBK115063.

Website Cuimhne Project and selected Irish dementia services

Cuimhne Irish Memory Loss Alliance: www.irishinbritain.org/what-we-do/our-campaigns/cuimhne-irish-memory-loss-alliance

Irish Community Services, Greenwich, Bexley and Lewisham: www.irishcommunityservices.org

Irish Community Care (Merseyside): http://iccm.org.uk

Leeds Irish Health and Homes: www.lihh.org

CHAPTER 3

Dementia and the UK African-Caribbean Community

David Truswell

The historical relationship between the UK and the Caribbean

The African-Caribbean community has a long-standing relationship with the UK, playing a central role since 1640 in the development of the economic power of the British Empire as a result of the chattel slavery of Africans transported to the Caribbean.

While the presence of African-Caribbean peoples in the UK is long-standing through this association with the trade in slaves, with the abolition of slavery and the subsequent colonial status of the Caribbean islands, the flow of migration from the Caribbean to the UK has persisted. This has been fuelled by push factors, such as the limited economic opportunities in the islands as the colonial power drained resources and capital from the economies, and pull factors, such as the participation of the young men and women from the Caribbean in the World War I and II and the 1950's post-war reconstruction in the UK.

The latter half of the 20th century saw significant increases in the numbers of people from the Caribbean, either as a consequence of coming to the UK during World War II or participating in the post-war economic recovery of the UK. The UK government of the 1950s made considerable efforts to recruit labour from the Caribbean to support the UK post-war recovery in a wide variety of industries and public services, emphasising in its appeal to Caribbean people a cultural commonality and the historical-cultural ties between the Caribbean and British cultures.

The immediate post-war period of Caribbean migration is usually referred to in UK mainstream media as the 'Windrush generation'. This is often presented as a static and sentimentalised caricature portraying the relationship between the Caribbean and UK as starting with the arrival of bemused Caribbean migrants on the *Empire Windrush* ship in 1948. This caricature glosses over the dynamic and historically fraught relationship going back hundreds of years between the former colonies and the UK, and the diverse and particular island identities of those from the Caribbean and of Caribbean descent. In the context of reminiscence work, a psychological return to childhood for those born in the Caribbean is to a particular island culture, where local terms, words and personal styles mark out the Jamaican, Bajan, Antiguan, Trinidadian and other island identities. Recall of the memory of arrival in the UK may also trigger much pain and trauma that may have been psychologically pushed aside for most of the individual's adult life.

Health risks, health inequity and the UK African-Caribbean community

International research on the health of migrant communities in developed countries has shown that there are a number of areas where migrant populations are commonly at more risk of developing illness than the mainstream population (International Organisation for Migration 2015). For the African-Caribbean population, there is a known increased risk of hypertension (Chaturvedi 2003). This elevates the risk of stroke and also the risk of vascular dementia, which it is estimated is an outcome of 20 per cent of cases of stroke (Tatemichi *et al.* 1992). The African-Caribbean population also has a raised risk of diabetes (Pitts-Tucker 2012), which researchers are increasingly linking with the risk of developing Alzheimer's disease (Sridhar, Lakshmi and Nagamani 2015). Research in the US on African Americans (Manly and Mayeux 2004) and in the UK on African-Caribbean population increasingly suggests that there is an increased risk of dementia in migrant populations of African descent, although there is insufficient research to allow any clear comparison between the dementia rate in the African diaspora and dementia rates in the countries of origin.

Issues with limitations in the quality of ethnicity recording in primary care and also in NHS hospital admission statistics further complicate an understanding of the increased risk of dementia in the African-Caribbean population in the UK (Pham *et al.* 2018). In its report, *Dementia does not discriminate*, the All-Party Parliamentary Group on Dementia (2013) estimated there would be a seven-fold increase in the number of people from BAME communities living with dementia by 2050, compared with an expected doubling of the numbers living with dementia in the White UK majority. Taking into account census data on the age structure of the UK minority communities, the current author (Truswell 2013) looked in more detail at individual ethnicity categories in the 2011 census and identified that much of this general increase in numbers of those living with dementia was experienced in the oldest settled minority communities in the UK – the Irish, Indian and African-Caribbean – rather than equally distributed across all minority communities. More recent data has suggested that in developed countries the global trend in increasing numbers of people living with dementia may be reaching a plateau or even declining (Prince *et al.* 2016). However, there is no evidence that any fine-grain analysis has been undertaken to determine if there is any similar decline in the increase in dementia rates in the BAME communities in the UK or in migrant communities in other developed countries.

While the broad risk factors of hypertension, coronary heart disease and diabetes are becoming much more robustly established as a general feature in understanding the risk profile for dementia of the African-Caribbean community and those of African-Caribbean descent, in the UK there is still limited clarity on the clinical implications of these broad risks. For example, while it is established that there is an increased risk of early onset dementia in the African-Caribbean community, some research speculation suggests that this involves a significant genetic component that differentiates this from later onset vascular dementia as a result of stroke (Kalaria *et al.* 2008). Similarly, the link between stroke risk and vascular dementia as a result of stroke is often cited as a generalised explanation for the increased rate of dementia in the African-Caribbean community (Adelman *et al.* 2011) but has not actually been demonstrated and confirmed in any large-scale research study, despite being strongly indicated in some smaller scale studies. There is little national-level work to develop any programme of targeted health education and preventative work with the African-Caribbean community (Jeraj and Butt 2018), despite the fact that this population is at significantly higher risk and that vascular dementia risk is reducible through diet and lifestyle changes that would reduce the risk of stroke.

'Black people don't get dementia' and 'Black communities look after their own'

Two pervasive and pernicious myths that are shared by many in the African-Caribbean community as well as those in the professional health and care services are that people from an African-Caribbean background have less risk of dementia (Berwald *et al.* 2016) than those in the White UK community and that traditional kinship expectations in African-Caribbean communities will lead families to provide for the bulk of the care and support needs of any family members who do develop dementia. Taken together, these beliefs can lead to people in the African-Caribbean community being reluctant to seek help and advice from primary care when they notice any signs of significant behavioural change that may be the early warning signs of dementia, and to the professional services either discounting or minimising these warning signs when they are reported to them by relatives and partners of patients. Professional services often presume a level of willingness and ability on the part of family carers from BAME communities to provide continuing support for the person showing early sign of living with dementia that is based on stereotyping of BAME communities.

It is only very recently that mainstream media information and depictions of people living with dementia have included images of people from the African-Caribbean communities and there are few stories of living with dementia articulated by people from these communities (Watson and *FT* readers 2017). Dementia is presented in the mainstream as largely an illness of White people, which leads to many people in African-Caribbean communities not being aware of the increased risk factors particular to their community.

The claim that 'families look after their own' does not consider how changes in longevity in developing countries, as they become increasingly comparable with longevity in developed countries, might impact on cultural expectations of care giving in later life. This is true of the African-Caribbean community and many others.

In the 1950s, when many of the then working-age or younger African-Caribbean migrants of the 'Windrush generation' came to the UK, the average lifespan in the Caribbean was 51.5 years. In the UK, by 2012 the average life span was 81, compared with an average lifespan in the Caribbean of 74 years (Department of Economic and Social Affairs 2012). Given the impact of lifetime economic impoverishment on the health of the population and a colonially under-resourced healthcare infrastructure in the post-war Caribbean, subsequently being depleted of its best and brightest to build the newly formed UK NHS of that period, it is unlikely that people routinely lived long enough at that point in the Caribbean to be subject to the age-related risks of dementia. They would have been more likely to die relatively early of the other health issues that are the common consequence of the mass poverty and hardship characterising underdeveloped colonial regimes.

Thus African-Caribbean people may have had less dementia in the Caribbean in the 1950s, as, in common with those in many other under-developed communities until very recently, people did not live long enough to enter the over-75 age range when the age-related risk of late-onset dementia starts to rise steeply. The misperception that African-Caribbean people are at less risk of dementia, rather than enhanced risk, has also been held by some people in clinical services, based on their observation that they do not see many people from African-Caribbean communities coming forward to seek assessment and help with early signs and symptoms. This under-representation in services is now being explored in clinical research, and barriers to presentation and access to services are gradually being better appreciated (Department of Economic and Social Affairs 2012).

Carers of people living with dementia have argued that caring for someone living with dementia is the most demanding form of caring. Many people with dementia have other significant health issues that require ongoing treatment, and the task of caring is likely to be psychologically distressing due to the personality changes in the person being cared for. The carer may themselves may be elderly with multiple health issues of their own to manage and they may be isolated from other potential support networks within their own community. Many carers have multiple caring obligations involving other dependents (Hill 2017).

Communities may have a general cultural familiarity with caring for elders, framed by historical experience in the country of origin where extended family members were physically close neighbours and recruiting additional support was easier through culturally shared expectations in the neighbourhood. However, the experience of migration and the globalisation of the families' experience through migration in the 20th/21st century provides new challenges to the inherited cultural narrative. It is not uncommon for contemporary multi-generational Caribbean families to be dispersed across the UK, US, Europe and the Caribbean. Even where children live in the same country as their elderly parents, they are likely to be geographically separated by significant distances. The physical distance separating potential family carers and the family member living with dementia may mean the burden of care falls on one family carer, who may feel thrust into the role as a result of location rather than choice.

It should not be assumed that even if the individual caring for the person living with dementia has previous experience of being a carer they feel competent to provide care or would make the choice to be the sole carer. People living with Alzheimer's disease may be ill and live with the significant impact of symptoms for 10–15 years, and with general population health improvement a higher proportion of those living with dementia will live longer with the disease. It is hardly credible that some hypothetical 'cultural familiarity' exists that ensures people will know how to cope as a sole carer supporting someone for years with a very complicated and psychologically challenging illness when the culture itself has little historical experience of this illness. This mythologised presumption that carers of those living with dementia in BAME communities can be simply left to 'look after their own' has no place as a default expectation in contemporary health policy in the UK.

Stigma, self-reliance and other barriers to seeking help

While the research evidence is very limited at this point, there is some emerging clarity regarding the role that stigma plays in inhibiting access to support from services and also in isolating the person living with dementia, and their carers, from support from other family members and more often the wider African-Caribbean community. Apart from the tendency to minimise the early signs of dementia or apparent increasing cognitive difficulties as just a sign of someone getting old, there is long-standing stigma within the African-Caribbean community regarding mental health issues. However, a great deal of work has been accomplished in the last 20 years in attempting to reduce this stigma (Carlotta *et al.* 2010) and some of the associated myths about people living with mental health problems.

Dementia is more likely to be viewed as a mental health issue by people in the African-Caribbean community and shares the stigma associated with mental health issues. Thus, the cultural narratives that identify dementia as a type of 'mental illness' rather than a physical disease of the brain also see dementia as having the same origins that are culturally ascribed to 'mental illness' – that is, they are caused by some family taint or 'bad blood' or by some demonic action, such as a curse, 'evil eye' or some form of demonic possession (Mantovani, Pizzolati and Edge 2016). The stigma discourages acknowledgement of early signs and symptoms and help-seeking outside the family and may lead people to seek support from more culturally appropriate figures to help with the perceived 'demons' and/or recourse to traditional practices or medicines or faith-based interventions.

However, stigma should not be taken as the sole explanation for people with the early signs and symptoms of dementia being reluctant to seek help from mainstream services. The culturally new experience of increasing levels of people living with dementia as longevity increases in all communities means there are more people around living with an illness that few people in the community understand. Many people simply do not know what to do. This means remedying the lack of information on how to recognise early signs and symptoms and challenging the notion that these are just a consequence of natural ageing. More could be done to improve the general public's understanding of the local diagnostic process and pathway through primary care. Community agencies such as traditional healers, the church and other faith groups could be helped to get practical information about service access better disseminated within the community or to provide awareness-raising within their own communities.

The experience of racial discrimination was strongly institutionalised to the point of being culturally normative in the 1950s in the UK, with the specific expressions of racist characterisation and hostility to those of African origin having roots back to the slavery period. Not confined to rooming house signs indicating 'No dogs, no Blacks, no Irish', this played out in 'race riots' and other smaller-scale acts of violence, intimidation and marginalisation that would have been familiar to many of the 'Windrush generation' through the early 1950s and 1960s. UK NHS mental health services have a poor record of their mental health service treatment of African-Caribbean patients that is long-standing and well researched, involving excessive force, over-medication and poor access to non-pharmacological treatments (Keating *et al.* 2002). Thus, the fear of experiencing discrimination to the point of fearing being physically at risk also contributes to making people reluctant to make contact with dementia services. As many UK dementia services are either located on mental health services sites or are functionally part of local mental health services, they share some of the anxious anticipation of an experience of discrimination and lack of cultural competence that is expected from these services by those from the African-Caribbean community.

The author has spoken to a number of first-generation African-Caribbean migrants of the Windrush generation and their carers at dementia awareness-raising events in the African-Caribbean community, as part of the work of the charity Culture Dementia UK, and this has highlighted a further factor contributing to the reluctance to seek help. This is the tradition of self-reliance and minimising of health issues, often expressed most strongly by Black men. Faced with the experience of discrimination and the limited opportunities available from the point of migration and onwards through a lifetime experience of socio-economic struggle, the first-generation migrant has a personal resilience and reliance on their own resources that has enabled survival and success and necessitated and embedded a reluctance to discuss any difficulties, including health problems, with colleagues, family or GPs.

There is a complex relationship between cultural beliefs about dementia, cultural fears of experiencing discrimination from services, cultural emphasis on self-reliance and independence, and cultural stereotyping by the service providers. This contributes to leaving the African-Caribbean community in the UK greatly underserved by current dementia research and dementia clinical support services and under-informed about risk and possible preventative action, despite being nationally one of the most at-risk groups for the vascular form of dementia.

A remedy for this state of affairs requires a more sophisticated approach than a single 'raising awareness' campaign or an isolated 'cultural competency' training initiative in a single site or service. A more useful approach can be found in work by authors such as Kenning *et al.* (2017), who advocate a 'two-pronged approach' incorporating community awareness-raising and education programmes for clinical staff being delivered in parallel (Kenning 2017). The current author has argued for improved understanding about how cultural beliefs and values impact on the experience of BAME communities across the whole pathway from initial seeking of a diagnosis to end-of-life care. A more fruitful research perspective would be that advocated by Zubair and Norris (2015), which emphasises the need to stop treating the migrant communities as the marginalised 'other' in research and service development programmes and bring community organisations into the research design structure.

Understanding the personal experience of people in the African–Caribbean community living with dementia

Every individual living through the experience of dementia will have a different experience that reflects who they are and their personal history.

Individual experience is unlikely to be reducible to a cultural template or cultural checklist that gives the provider of care a cast-iron assurance that they must be doing everything well if they tick all the correct boxes. At the individual level, the disease itself is corrosive of assurance and certainty as the person living with dementia no longer lives in a world of being sure of themselves or their experiences, and family carers lose their sense of assurance about who they are caring for.

Demographic projections indicate that the numbers of people in the African-Caribbean population living with dementia will rise far more steeply than in the majority White population over the next 30 years. Understanding of dementia risk within the African-Caribbean population is poor and research on this high-risk community is very limited, with few targeted interventions such as targeted information campaigns, increasing recruitment from this population into research programmes, increasing diagnostic rates and earlier diagnosis. Recent joint work involving Public Health England, the Race Equality Foundation, the Dementia Alliance for Culture and Ethnicity and a number of community organisations has been an exception to this, with a short series of events across England from November 2017 to March 2018 (Jeraj and Butt, 2018).

Developing appropriate support interventions, for example culturally appropriate reminiscence materials for a different community, only exists in the form of a few isolated, time-limited pilot studies with low numbers of participants. Some useful materials have been developed from work by a number of community groups or associations that cover a variety of different ethnic communities, such as Chinese National Healthy Living Centre, Irish in Britain, Ekta, Alzheimer's Society, Liverpool Dementia Action Alliance and Meri Yaadain. A number of third-sector organisations nationally have built a considerable body of experience in working with dementia in the African-Caribbean communities, such as Dementia Alliance for Culture and Ethnicity, Dementia UK, Culture Dementia UK, Nubian Life and Pearl Support Network. The dementia research community needs to more actively reach out to organisations such as these and develop working partnerships.

There is a strong cultural tradition of respect for elders in the African-Caribbean community, which adds to the discomfort of holding any community discourse about dementia since this involves facing up to the idea of respected elders losing mental faculties and their capacity for self-reliance.

Mothers, fathers and partners who have been the immovable rocks of a carer's life may be seen to be crumbling in the face of the onset of dementia. Lifetime economic and social discrimination contribute to the financial challenges of supporting elders living with dementia, and family carers who cannot provide direct care may themselves directly finance paid carers. Often family carers will find themselves expected to be the cultural expert for the provider organisation and have to pay supplementary costs to meet the cultural needs of the person living with dementia. Work done in the US on the supplementary costs of dementia support by family carers for African Americans indicates that these can be considerable (Gaskin, LaVeist and Richard 2013).

There is little evident consideration in the literature of these supplementary costs, which may, for example, extend to hair and skin care products, appropriate leisure activities, and end-of-life provision. The costs may be considerable over the duration of time spent with illness. In practice, this may mean that family carers act as unacknowledged subsidisers of the statutory service, allowing the service to evade examining its own systemic practice shortcomings in providing dementia care appropriate to a diverse community.

A stereotypical assumption is that the family carer in the African-Caribbean community will be supported by their local faith community and that national generic faith initiatives encouraging support for those living with dementia will be taken up by the African-Caribbean faith communities. While Christian ministry and the Christian Church often play a significant role in supporting the cultural identity and providing a personal spiritual resource for those migrants of the Windrush generation, second generation offspring who may have key roles as family carers may have less connection with the same faith communities of their parents.

The degree to which these faith communities respond to supporting people living with dementia, and their carers, will be highly variable and the attitude of the local minister will be critical. The church can fail at the personal level of providing spiritual solace for the person living with dementia through the minister's lack of understanding of dementia or through the congregation not yet being ready to provide understanding or peer support to the family in an informed way. It is possible that for the individual living with dementia or a family carer, support from the physical place, ceremonies and texts of their faith are critical as a spiritual support, but at the same time they do not feel they can talk to their minister or anyone in their congregation about their dementia or the dementia of a family member. The role of both faith as a spiritual, personal resource and faith communities as social networks for support needs to be better understood in the context of the individual's situation and needs. The subtleties of the personal spiritual experience of being 'in/with my spirit' that some will refer to is not the same thing as the relationship with the local congregation.

Some individual experiences

A number of people from an African-Caribbean background with experience as carers or with living with dementia agreed to be interviewed for this book.

Ronald's story: Living with dementia

Ronald is a 59-year-old Jamaican man. Nearly three years after being hospitalised as a result of a stroke, Ronald was diagnosed with 'mixed dementia', both vascular dementia and Alzheimer's disease. Ronald's mother died with vascular dementia when she was in her eighties. He thinks it is time the African-Caribbean community started learning more about dementia and talking about how to get help rather than trying to 'tough it out'.

He knows a thing or two about 'toughing it out'. Ronald left school at 13 and spent the next few years graduating through reform school and youth offender custody to a prison sentence. It was when he was out of prison that his sister took him along to a recording studio. The visit was organised by Janet Kaye, a hugely popular reggae singer at the time and also a friend of Ronald's sister. For Ronald, who says he could see he was 'on his way down' at this time, it was the start of a major turnaround of his life as he got to know more about the music business and understood that he could make something of his life through music.

He started to learn about music production and knuckle down to the hard work needed to make a successful living out of writing music, producing and managing. At one point he ran a popular local night club and also was giving back to the community through working with youth caught up in the criminal 'fast life' to help them develop confidence and get out. While his career in music completely changed his life, Ronald is not sentimental about the music business, recognising that developing and sustaining a career in the business also needed toughness.

When he started having problems with being reliable about appointments and meeting commitments and increasingly losing his patience with people, he dismissed it as 'stress'. He had previously been having problems with his neck for a couple of years. He decided this was also 'stress'. In response, Ronald did what most African-Caribbean men usually do with any health issue; he ignored it and 'toughed it out'. When he started to forget things or found people were complaining that he had done things he could not remember doing, he 'toughed it out'. He wasn't going to see a doctor. He says, 'I knew something was wrong, but I was in denial. If someone said I'd done something, and I couldn't remember, I just got angry. I wouldn't have it.'

He carried on 'toughing it out', until three years ago when he collapsed at home, alone. Despite lying on the floor with his phone, telling the emergency operator that he thought he was dying, he somehow managed to drag himself across the room to open the door to let the ambulance driver in. He says he has no idea how he was able to do it. He had a further stroke while in hospital.

While Ronald still has plenty of challenges in his life, he has found that the best thing for keeping his own motivation and positive attitude is listening to music. He has embarked on a music project disseminated on social media, continues to make music, is mentoring a singer, writes poetry and has been working with Culture Dementia UK and the Dementia Alliance for Culture and Ethnicity to raise awareness about dementia in the African-Caribbean community through talking and writing about his experience.

Julie's story: Living with dementia

Julie had to recognise that the problems she was having with her memory were getting serious when her 12-year-old grandson pointed out, 'Nanny, you keep forgetting.' When she asked him what it was he thought she forgot, his reply was, 'You forget everything.' His sister agreed.

Julie is a woman in her early fifties who was born in the Dominican Republic. She works as the chief executive officer of a user-led national charity in the UK that she founded and developed herself and has built up over the past 20 years to provide support, information and advice services to people with vulnerabilities. She has long-standing struggles with physical disabilities and mental health issues herself, yet has worked hard to ensure that the charity is highly regarded and has herself been a ministerial advisor for some years. She lost her mother in 2017 as a result of a catastrophic storm in Dominica that destroyed the family home.

Normally a very organised woman, Julie had begun to have problems with her memory before the loss of her mother. Her mother had been providing her with some personal support before she left the UK to return to the family home in Dominica in 2017. The category 8 storm in September 2017 took away the breadfruit tree that had grown in the garden when it swept away the entire house and led to the loss of her mother's life. Julie describes returning to the family home in the aftermath as 'like seeing that all my memories had been ripped away and there was nothing left'. The period surrounding the funeral and the return to the UK she describes as a 'complete blank'.

Previously at ease with addressing conference audiences and speaking to senior health and care officials, she now feels a lot of her confidence has been lost. Her phone is a lifeline, allowing her to organise her daily life, but in many ways managing a lot of the tasks of daily living is compromised. Sticky-style memory notes don't work for her because she loses the notes. She feels unable to open mail as she feels that the information will prove to be too complex and confusing. Although separated from her partner, there are joint financial matters that need to be resolved from their relationship that she feels unable to face. While Julie has the support of a paid carer due to her pre-existing disability challenges, she is concerned that the carer may not be the right person to support her with her financial issues.

Julie talked to her GP for the first time about her worries about her increasing forgetfulness a few months ago. While the GP had indicated that the next move was a referral to a memory clinic, there has been no further contact or advice about managing the symptoms. A call to the GP surgery on the day of the interview with the author revealed that there was no indication in the medical notes that the referral letter had yet been sent. Julie feels that her memory has continued to decline since she spoke to the GP a few months ago. She feels she is also getting more irritable and suspicious with people.

Julie is living with a recent bereavement and marital breakdown as well as managing her ongoing personal health issues. She is conscientiously trying to continue doing her job but when she is not absent through being too ill to work, her memory has become unreliable. Her GP's preliminary view is this may be the onset of early dementia, but little advice has been given on information to help with managing the current symptoms and there seems a lack of urgency about the referral process to memory services.

Julie needs urgent help with her financial issues and would like some personal support time through either a befriender or a daytime resource service. Lasting Power of Attorney was discussed in the interview with the author and this was the first time this had been proposed to her.

Sharron's story: A carer's perspective

Sharron is a civil servant. Her father is in the early stages of dementia; the diagnosis was only confirmed recently but her mother has been saying for some time that something was happening to him. Sharron decided about 18 months ago they needed to take him to the doctor. They did some initial short tests but found nothing wrong with his memory. Her mother and father have been married for 50 years but what her mother had first noticed wasn't a change in his memory but in his personality. He had always been a pretty easy-going man, but he started to become irritable and aggressive, although not violent.

Getting him to go to see the doctor was hard work. Sharron had to tell him it was about his hypertension to get him to go. She went in with him for the memory tests and feels they were pretty inappropriate and culturally invalid – hardly the sort of things her dad could be expected to know. At the first visit, the GP was a locum who didn't even know her dad and who spoke with a pronounced accent that was hard to understand. The memory test questions were about things like WWI and WWII and she had thought, 'How is my dad expected to know this?' She felt she had to 'interpret' and rephrase the questions to make sense of them for her father.

Now his memory problems seem to come and go. More recently, for example, he can't remember what he had for breakfast. One good thing about the first memory tests was that when they went back to see the GP again some time later as the problems were getting worse, at least the GP had a baseline score to compare the more recent scores to, and this helped to get a referral to Croydon Memory Service. Her mother and father are very positive about the service, they feel listened to and the staff there get the whole family's view on her father's problems. It was also important to her mother that there was another Black person in the assessment team for the diagnosis and that the team will come to the house to discuss the next steps.

Sharron's mum hasn't told Sharron's brothers and sisters yet, and Sharron is encouraging her to let them know that they need to recognise that their mother needs support too; her father also needs to recognise this. When she lived in St Lucia, her mother had an aunt who had dementia. Her mother remembers when she went back to St Lucia some years ago with her husband to visit her aunt, her aunt could remember her but not her husband, even though the aunt had known both of them since their childhood.

Sharron feels that they have known there was something going on with her father for some time but even with the diagnosis it's still taking a while to digest. She recently went on holiday with her parents back to St Lucia and visited her father's family. Her father was really animated when they came back, and while he was away he had a great time being with his brothers reminiscing. He is the oldest of his siblings. She feels it is important to keep him socially engaged and active. He always has been a very active man – until recently he used to do at least 50 push-ups every day but then he had a shoulder injury. She has been trying to get him to take up Tai Chi.

Sharron would like to see more done to encourage families to be more aware of the possible symptoms of dementia and to look for help before they get too severe. In her own family, her siblings don't all have the same view of what is happening to their father. Her brother, for example, carries on saying he's fine because he does not see him often enough to recognise what he is going through. For her, the first real sign of a change in her father was four years ago when everyone got together at Christmas and in the middle of everyone chatting away and the music playing her father suddenly blew up and started complaining about the noise. This was completely unlike him as he was usually in his element with the talking and the music. She feels that people need to understand dementia isn't only about memory loss, and sometimes an early sign might be when someone who is close to you shows a change in their usual behaviour that persists over a period. She also feels that dementia professionals need to talk to people close to the person living with dementia to better understand their personality and behaviour changes.

Linda's story: A carer's perspective

Linda is a widow who describes her age as '25 plus VAT'. She is bringing up her son as a single parent while working as a civil servant. Born and brought up in North London by her Caribbean parents, she studied at the School of Oriental and African Studies and worked as an optician before finding herself in the civil service. Her father has recently passed away after living with dementia for many years.

Linda recalls that despite the many paid carers her father had during his illness, she could always easily tell the difference between the ones who only did the job for the money and those who developed a genuine relationship with her dad. These were the ones he was always pleased to see. Linda herself was very seriously ill at one stage while her father was bedbound with dementia. She was discharged from hospital to her parent's home and she had an opportunity then to see at first-hand all the help he received from the paid carers as well as play an increasing role as a carer for him herself. She feels that as a dementia carer you end up having to 'be a parent to the parent'. She feels that GPs, dementia professionals and paid carers needed to know how to speak to her dad otherwise he would not respond. Rather than just ask him stupid questions they should talk to him about things he was interested in like cricket, dominoes and food.

Her parents waited ten years before they had her, so as she was growing up her parents were much older than her friends' parents. Now she is finding more and more that the friends she grew up with are having to come to terms with having a parent who is living with dementia, so she can talk with them and understand what they are going through and share her experience.

Looking back now, she thinks there were a couple of key points in the period before her father was diagnosed that stick in her mind as indicators that something was happening with her father. Her parents loved a programme on Sky TV called *Maury* and one day she visited them while the show was on in the background. Her dad took a stool and went over and sat by the TV and when one of the characters on the screen left the set, her dad started tapping on the top of the TV. When she asked what he was doing, he explained he was trying to get the character who had left to come back onto the screen.

A second key moment happened when her father left the house, telling her mother he was just going to the local shop. By 6pm, three hours later, he had not returned. They called the police. A short time later, her father came walking down the road with a local neighbour who had found him wandering in a nearby park, some distance from the shops that had been his intended destination. He explained he had been going towards the school to find out where his kids were as they had not come back from school after he had taken them there in the morning. Linda and her siblings are all adults. At a later stage, her father began hoarding things in plastic bags and would not let people examine the bags. He also started to claim that various items belonging to him were going missing.

Linda's father was lucky enough to have a good long-standing relationship with his GP, who would visit him at home from time to time. Her father eventually died with severe constipation and she had to learn that this was a common problem in dementia. In the early stages, her mother did not recognise dementia and felt he was just being 'a miserable old goat'. Linda feels that perhaps the darkest time of her father living with dementia was in the period before he got the diagnosis, which lasted about four years, when they struggled to understand his changed behaviour. When she went to see him with her late husband, he would not recognise her husband even though he had known him since he was a child. However, her father always seemed to be aware that he had a granddaughter.

He was living at home and going to a Caribbean day-care service twice a week and this was all working well until her father had a fall at home. When the ambulance service arrived, they felt that it would be best to take him to hospital for a fuller check-up. He had been taking Aricept, which had been helping to keep him calm, but there was some mix-up about his medication and the hospital stopped it. He became confused and deteriorated, at one point being found curled up on the floor in a foetal position. He was moved into a rehabilitation unit and, having walked in there using a Zimmer frame, became bedbound in the unit and never walked again. The unit finally admitted that there was a mix-up with his medication and wanted to transfer him to a nursing home as they claimed he was becoming aggressive and difficult to manage.

The family refused to have him moved into a nursing home and made arrangements for him to return home for his care. With support from the GP, occupational health and visiting carers, Linda's father continued to live at home for a further three years before he died. The support provided included two paid carers visiting four times a day. Linda feels that this was the best care he could have had.

When her father had additional carer support in the earlier period of living with dementia, he refused to have female carers but this changed when he got towards the stage of needing more intimate personal care and he did not want a male carer for this. Because her mum and dad were both proud people, things got difficult when Linda's father reached the point when he was doubly incontinent. An incident that stands out for her was when her mum was in tears because her dad had 'messed himself' and she couldn't clean the house before the carers turned up. Linda describes how her mother would tidy up and her father would struggle to wash and shave himself to make sure they were presentable for the carer's arrival. It took a long time for them to get used to accepting that the carers were coming to do the washing, shaving and personal care for them. Her parents were very self-conscious about strangers coming into the house.

After her experience, Linda feels that people living with dementia need a good GP and a strong family to support them because there needs to be people around who are willing to fight for them. In the end, her father died in her mother's arms after saying the Lord's Prayer with her, and he knew who his family were right up to the end.

Concluding summary

African-Caribbean identity is heterogenous, often linked to the history and culture of a specific island, with reminiscence and memory tied intimately to place for first-generation migrants. Stories shared between older migrants evoke a sense of a time and place shared between them while their children who have grown up in the UK may not have had similar childhood experiences. Individual history and personal resilience can play a strong part in the reluctance of African-Caribbean people to ask for help when this is viewed as an unacceptable admission of vulnerability. Many African-Caribbean people are not aware of the higher risk factors for dementia in the African-Caribbean community and much more sustained and culturally relevant dementia awareness-raising needs to be focused on this community. While stigma has a role in the reluctance to seek help with dementia, the psychological and cultural components of this reluctance are complex and interact with institutional stereotyping by services. Working with the family is often key to both initial and sustained engagement with dementia services. Working with the person as an individual must include working with the historical and cultural understanding they have of themselves and how this is expressed by them throughout the development of their dementia. The personal stories in this chapter show how personal independence and competence dynamically interact with areas of incapacity and vulnerability in the myriad adjustments to dealing with needing support and care.

Reminiscence can trigger recall of traumatic life events linked to the historic experience of racism, which perhaps have for a lifetime been kept under emotional wraps. Carers and family members struggle not only with the loss of parents, spouses or parental figures but those same figures can have been the primary bulwark and reference point in their lives against a hostile environment. The same figures may now reveal unimagined vulnerabilities or exhibit incomprehensible behaviours as they live with the progress of the disease.

Information that presents the experience of dementia through the lens of the African-Caribbean community is rare, although there is some improvement with mainstream media representation including people from the African-Caribbean community living with dementia, and their carers, speaking out. Support for carers may be hit and miss, with faith organisations or community groups in some local instances being extremely helpful. Similarly, the quality of support from statutory organisations across the pathway from GP surgery to memory clinics and on to community social care and residential care can be a lottery. In personal testimonies, many of those telling their stories can highlight examples of both very good and sensitive help and bad practice and incompetence. Professional care is delivered in silos that rarely connect up.

Good practice can rely heavily on a single dedicated practitioner and risks collapsing if that individual is sick or moves on. Despite the higher and yet modifiable risk factors for vascular dementia for the African-Caribbean population, research work, with a very few notable exceptions, has barely begun.

There needs to be much more robust action at the research and commissioning level to identify the scale of risk in the African-Caribbean population at the locality level and to develop local services to both meet the awareness-raising and preventive aspect of the agenda and provide an appropriate supporting structure through the dementia pathway from pre-diagnostic publicity to end-of-life care for this population. This action should include mobilising the sustainable support of social networks such as faith groups and community groups to play a significant role, along with family carers where these are available. At present, the failure to take this action all too often leaves families at risk of taking the burden of trying to secure adequate care and support entirely on their own shoulders, with their loved one's labelled as 'difficult' when they suffer the disabling consequences of poor and culturally uninformed institutional care.

References

Adelman, S., Blanchard, M., Greta Rai, G., Leavey, G. and Livingston, G. (2011) 'Prevalence of dementia in African–Caribbean compared with UK-born White older people: Two-stage cross-sectional study.' *The British Journal of Psychiatry,* 198, 1–7.

All Party Parliamentary Group on Dementia (2013) *Dementia does not discriminate: The experiences of black, Asian and minority ethnic communities.* London: All Party Parliamentary Group on Dementia.

Berwald, S., Roche, M., Adelman, S., Mukadam, N. and Livingston, G. (2016) 'Black African and Caribbean British communities' perceptions of memory problems: "We don't do dementia".' *PLoS, ONE,* 11, 4: e0151878. doi:10.1371/journal.pone.0151878.

Carlotta, A., Hickling, F., Robertson-Hickling, H. Haynes-Robinson, T., Wendel, A. and Whitley, R. (2010) '"Mad, sick, head nuh good": Mental illness stigma in Jamaican communities.' *Transcultural Psychiatry,* 47, 252–275.

Chaturvedi, N. (2003) 'Ethnic differences in cardiovascular disease.' *Heart,* 89, 6:681–686.

Department of Economic and Social Affairs (2012) *Population Facts No. 2012/2.* United Nations Population Division.

Gaskin, D., LaVeist, T. and Richard, P. (2013) *The Costs of Alzheimer's and Other Dementia for African Americans.* African American Network Against Alzheimer's.

Hill, A. (2017) 'Hidden carers: The sixty-somethings looking after parents and grandchildren.' *The Guardian* (Monday 13 February 2017).

International Organisation for Migration (2015) *World Migration Report 2015: Migrants and Cities: New Partnerships to Manage Mobility*. Geneva: International Organisation for Migration.

Jeraj, S. and Butt, J. (2018) *Dementia and Black, Asian and Minority Ethnic Communities. Report of a Health and Wellbeing Alliance Project*. VSCE Health and Wellbeing Alliance. Available at: http://raceequalityfoundation.org.uk/wp-content/uploads/2018/09/ Dementia-and-BAME-Communities-report-Final-v2.pdf.

Kalaria, R., Maestre, G, Arizaga R., Friedland, R. P. *et al.* (2008) *Alzheimer's disease and vascular dementia in developing countries: prevalence, management, and risk factors*. Available at: www.thelancet.com/neurology Published online 28 July 2008. doi:10.1016/S1474-4422(08)70169-8y.

Keating, K., Robertson, D., McCulloch, and Francis, E. (2002) *Breaking the Circles of Fear: A Review of the Relationship Between Mental Health Services and African and Caribbean Communities*. London: The Sainsbury Centre for Mental Health.

Kenning, C., Daker-White, G., Blakemore, A., Panagioti, M. and Waheed, W. (2017) 'Barriers and facilitators in accessing dementia care by ethnic minority groups: A meta-synthesis of qualitative studies.' *BMC Psychiatry*, 17, 316.

Manly, J. and Mayeux, R. (2004) 'Ethnic Differences in Dementia and Alzheimer's Disease.' In National Research Council (US) Panel on Race, Ethnicity, and Health in Later Life; N.B. Anderson, R.A. Bulatao and B. Cohen (eds) *Critical Perspectives on Racial and Ethnic Differences in Health in Late Life*. Washington, DC: National Academies Press.

Mantovani, N., Pizzolati, M. and Edge, D. (2016) 'Exploring the relationship between stigma and help-seeking for mental illness in African-descended faith communities in the UK.' *Health Expectations*, 20, 3, 373–384.

Pham, T.M., Petersen, P., Walters, K., Raine, R. *et al.* (2018) 'Trends in dementia diagnosis rates in UK ethnic groups: Analysis of UK primary care data.' *Epidemiology*, 10, 949–960.

Pitts-Tucker, T. (2012) 'Asian and Afro-Caribbean Britons have double the risk of type 2 diabetes.' *British Medical Journal*, 345: e6135.

Prince, M., Gemma-Claire, A., Maëlenn, G., Matthew, P.A. *et al.* (2016) 'Recent global trends in the prevalence and incidence of dementia, and survival with dementia.' *Alzheimers Research and Therapy*, 8, 1, 23.

Sridhar, G.R., Lakshmi, G. and Nagamani, G. (2015) 'Emerging links between Type 2 diabetes and Alzheimer's disease.' *World Journal of Diabetes*, 6, 5, 744–751.

Tatemichi, T., Desmond, D., Mayeux, P., Paik, M. *et al.* (1992) 'Dementia after stroke: Baseline frequency, risks, and clinical features in a hospitalized cohort.' *Neurology*, 42, 6, 1185–1193.

Truswell, D. (2013) *Black, Asian and Minority Ethnic Communities and Dementia – Where Are We Now?* Better Health Briefing Paper 30. London: Race Equality Foundation.

Watson, W. and *FT* readers (2017) 'Stories from the front line of dementia.' *The Financial Times* (20 December 2017).

Zubair, M. and Norris, M. (2015) 'Perspectives on ageing, later life and ethnicity: Ageing research in ethnic minority contexts.' *Ageing & Society*, 35, 5, 897–916.

CHAPTER 4

The Experience of Dementia in UK South Asian Communities

Dr Karan Jutlla and Harjinder Kaur

Introduction

In the 2001 census, South Asians were 3.9 per cent of the total UK population and by 2011 this figure had risen to 5.3 per cent. The 2011 UK census recorded 1,451,862 residents of Indian, 1,174,983 of Pakistani and 451,529 of Bangladeshi ethnicity, making a total South Asian population of 3,078,374, excluding other Asian groups and people of mixed ethnicity. Current estimations suggest that approximately 25,000 people from Black, Asian and minority ethnic (BAME) communities in the UK are living with dementia (All Party Parliamentary Group on Dementia 2013). However, the true prevalence of dementia within the UK South Asian community is yet to be established (Blakemore *et al.* 2018). Nonetheless, the growing South Asian population in the UK means that the prevalence of dementia in these communities will increase.

The challenges and barriers faced by South Asian communities in the UK when caring for a person with dementia have been well documented. Several studies (Jolley *et al.* 2009; Jutlla 2013, 2015; Jutlla and Moreland 2007, 2009; Moriarty, Sharif and Robinson 2011; Seabrooke and Milne 2004) remind us that, generally, South Asian communities have poor knowledge and understanding of dementia and what it involves, predominantly because there is no word for 'dementia' in any of the South Asian languages (Hindi, Punjabi, Urdu, Gujarati and Bangladeshi). Consequently, dementia is often conceptualised as a mental health problem rather than a neurological disorder, thus bringing with it the stigma attached to such illnesses. Due to this stigma, dementia can often remain hidden in such communities, with those in need of support presenting themselves to services only when in crisis situations.

Evidence also suggests that dementia is sometimes viewed as a normal part of the ageing process and some even understand symptoms of dementia by religious belief (Kenning *et al.* 2017).

Furthermore, studies suggest that cultural norms within such communities can lead to a reluctance to ask for, and accept, formal support. For example, Jutlla (2011) found that cultural expectations around familial roles and a duty to care in the Sikh community often meant that carers refused support from services. Other studies have highlighted the need to portray an image of wellbeing to those outside the family (MacKenzie 2007). This, coupled with a general lack of knowledge and access to services, places such individuals in challenging situations. There are also assumptions about community support and that South Asian families tend to 'look after their own' (Department of Health 1998).

According to Blakemore and colleagues (2018), low levels of literacy, language barriers and a lack of appropriately translated and culturally adapted screening tools and diagnostic tools create challenges in diagnosing dementia in such communities. Though dementia diagnosis rates are low, there is evidence to suggest that vascular dementia is common due to higher incidences of hypertension, diabetes and stroke in these communities (All Party Parliamentary Group on Dementia 2013). Subsequently, those who do use services have suggested that they are culturally inappropriate due to cultural and language barriers (Regan 2014).

Although the challenges faced by such communities have been well documented, areas such as community perspectives of dementia, and the impact of migration warrant further exploration. We, the authors, draw on our experiences of research and education in this area (Karan Jutlla) and clinical expertise (Harjinder Kaur) to make suggestions for how people living with dementia, and their families, from South Asian communities in the UK can be better supported. Where appropriate, quotes have been taken from research with Sikh carers of a family member with dementia living in Wolverhampton (Jutlla 2011) and case examples have been taken from practice to illustrate our discussions. Pseudonyms have used to maintain confidentiality, and where necessary, attributes have been adapted.

Understanding dementia: community perspectives

Though there is, to an extent, poor knowledge and understanding of dementia in South Asian communities, the different conceptualisations around dementia warrant further exploration. Western versus eastern ideologies involve not only geographical differences but also differences in schools of thought. The main differences between the school of thought of the East and West are suggested to be the West's Individualism and the East's Collectivism. The eastern philosophy is drawn much more into groups or society or people's actions and thoughts as one in order to find meaning in life, whereas western philosophies are more individualistic, trying to find the meaning of life here and now, with self at the centre (Differences Between 2018). It could be suggested that one of the ways in which such collectivism is expressed is via language. In most South Asian cultures and languages, respect is given to people by referring to them as a relational role. For example, the community psychiatric nurse (CPN) was always 'daughter,' or 'sister' to a family in receipt of treatment. Similarly, they for her were all 'aunts, uncles, brothers and sisters'. Coming from South Asian descent ourselves, we know that referring to someone as a relational role implies recognition, respect and trust and says, 'we are all family – we are all connected'. In the Punjabi language, for example, where respect is to be given, references should always be made in the plural and never singular; so, if an elder is sleeping, we would always say 'they are asleep' and never 'she/he is asleep', as in Punjabi, the latter is how you would refer to younger people or friends. The point here is not to learn the language but rather to understand that notions of collectivism, togetherness, mutual respect and trust are built into South Asian communities. Such notions of collectivism are useful for understanding the ways in which dementia is conceptualised in such communities.

Indeed, research with South Asian carers of a person with dementia (Jutlla and Moreland 2007) and later, Sikh carers (Jutlla 2011), revealed that even those who have been educated on dementia understood it to be something concerned with a much bigger picture. Despite being told it is the destruction of brain cells, some people believed that the dementia developed as the result of migration, hard work, stressful activities, alienation, isolation and loneliness, and, in some cases, a preparation for end of life and an opportunity to do 'seva' (selfless service). Older Sikh migrants believed dementia was the breakdown of community norms and the mind naturally returning to a place where life was at its best – back home (Jutlla 2011); it was the result of a mind 'unfit' for western ways of living, which involved abandonment from children, isolation and loneliness.

We are not suggesting that dementia education serves no purpose in these communities but rather, it is important to have an understanding that for migrants from eastern parts of the world, there will be cultural variations in the way in which they conceptualise the information they are given. For example, Harbans Kaur, aged 70 years, cares for her husband who has dementia. When asked if she knew what dementia was, she stated:

> It is when the brain is not working. The brain starts to die in different places. But I'm not surprised. It's been a hard life in this country… working, raising children, educating them. He thinks he's back in Punjab most of the time, reliving the happiest years of his life. That time when everyone was together. You need your people to survive in this life, without them what is there?

Similarly, Darshan Kaur, aged 44 years and caring for her mother, stated:

> You know, I'm not surprised this (dementia) has happened to her. She came to a foreign country where she knew no one…gave birth to five girls. She then lost her husband and had to listen to her brothers all her life. So did we. None of my sisters married Indian men, only me. That's why she's okay staying with me. I guess she feels like she's got nothing in common with the world now. Why wouldn't she go back there (country of birth) in her mind?

What we, the authors, find most interesting about this is that, although there is a yearning for community cohesion, support and understanding, the stigma associated with dementia means that attempts are made to ensure that the outside community do not become aware of such circumstances. As mentioned earlier, because of the associated symptoms of dementia, it is often interpreted as a mental health illness. As with most communities, regardless of ethnicity, there is a stigma around mental health. Both the evidence base and our experiences of working with South Asian communities reveal not just the stigma of dementia but also, the consequent stigma of using services. For example, Simarjeet Kaur, a 49-year-old woman who cares for her mother, when informed of her financial entitlements, stated: 'I've never asked because they'll start saying…she's taking money for her mom. It's very expensive, they (Asians) don't realise…it's hard to get by' (cited in Jutlla 2014). A similar statement was made by Ranjit Kaur, aged 33 years, who cares for her father:

I really struggled at the beginning... Mainly because I wouldn't send dad to day care. I was scared of what the (Sikh) community would say about me for sending him... That I wasn't a good daughter... And that I couldn't look after him properly. But the CPN encouraged me to do it and although it really helps me because I work as well, I still feel that they are pointing fingers at me. It's horrible really...I feel like an outcast.

Though there is the common perception that people from South Asian families look after their own, the reasons for this are complex and quite often, such families need further support. One of us (Harjinder Kaur) has years of experience of working directly with South Asian families as their CPN and notes that upon the first visit, many family members will gather and often an assumption is made that strong informal support structures are in place. However, the day-to-day caring activities are usually taking place in isolation from other family members and it is important that services do not assume that further support is not required or necessary.

Furthermore, changes in lifestyle and work commitments mean that fewer families live together as extended families. Consequently, older people from South Asian communities are living alone, with many unable to access services due to challenges with literacy and English language ability. Even those who learned to speak English will at some point in their dementia revert to their mother tongue. Though there are collective community and cultural norms that influence help-seeking behaviours, it is important that a personalised approach is taken. Key to providing individualised care is understanding the person's life history. For South Asian communities in the UK, this includes their experiences of migration.

Dementia and migration

The impact of migration and migrant identities on experiences of caring for a family member with dementia and service use have been discussed (see Jutlla 2014). However, the impact of such experiences for a migrant living with dementia is an area seldom discussed in the literature. This is a very important issue when considering the South Asian communities living in the UK – especially as dementia can involve an associated rollback memory loss whereby the older memory can become more prominent.

As highlighted by Mackenzie (2007, p.76), to achieve 'mutually satisfying user/provider relationships such people should be regarded as individuals alongside knowledge of the social and political influences on their lives rather than regarding them as members of *"other"* groups.' Though there are cultural norms within South Asian communities that will influence both perceptions and decision making around dementia care, there are also political influences on migrants living in the UK. Many of the South Asian population now growing old in the UK have life experiences from key historical events such as the 1947 India and Pakistan partition, the 1982 Khalistan movement and many more. Furthermore, the UK in the 1960s was reported as a hostile environment to live in for migrants, many of whom suffered the consequences of direct racial attacks (James 1974). Such traumatic experiences are embedded in the emotional memory which, for people living with dementia, becomes the most prominent. For a person living with dementia, if a feeling of 'threat' occurs, the mind may recall a memory where a similar feeling arose. Because of the complexity of the dementia, the mind may be unable to distinguish that the recalled memory is a memory of the past and not the present moment. Let us share with you some examples from practice.

Randeep

Randeep Singh is 83 years old. He has vascular dementia and his wife is his main carer. They live alone together with their children close by. Randeep arrived in the UK in the 1960s for industrial work in Handsworth, alongside many others from India. This mass migration to the area had caused a political protest by the National Front who ran a series of violent attacks with the aim to send migrant communities back home. Like many others, Randeep stood by his South Asian migrant peers and fought for their right to stay in the UK. Randeep often spoke about these experiences with his wife and later his children too – to remind them that their place within the UK is one which was fought for.

Following Randeep's diagnosis, provisions for paid carers to help with personal hygiene were put in place by the CPN. Although there were several South Asian carers available, most of these were women. Understandably, Randeep stated that he would prefer a male care worker. Due to the dearth of South Asian male care workers, Randeep was assigned a White British carer to help him.

For the first three weeks, there were no problems. Randeep had established a good relationship with the carer and they seemed to get on well. However, one day Randeep's wife called the CPN as a matter of urgency. She informed the CPN that Randeep was becoming aggressive towards the carer and had reached a stage where he was starting to be physically violent towards him. She couldn't understand what had changed, and neither could the carer. With understandable concerns, Randeep's wife complained to the care supplier, claiming that the carer must be doing something to aggravate the situation. An investigation began and the CPN offered to speak with Randeep to see if she could put his behaviour into context and assess whether his condition was deteriorating.

Through lengthy conversations, the CPN discovered that Randeep understood the carer to be part of the National Front and therefore someone who was going to hurt him and attempt to get him out of his home. The change had occurred as a result of a television programme that Randeep had recently watched involving images of the National Front and the riots that had taken place. Quite often, the complexity of dementia can mean that some are unable to remember or recognise that television dramas are not reality and are witnessed and understood as a live, present situation. This is more so the case with flat screen televisions as a person of Randeep's age will recall televisions to be the box sets they were in the 1950s. A decision was made to change the male care worker to a White British female worker.

The important point here is that Randeep's condition had not deteriorated but was influenced by an external situation which caused him to recall traumatic events in his own life. Indeed then, the appearance of a White British male trying to get close to him brought feelings of threat and anxiety for Randeep. Abdul, too, reminds us of a case example where migration experiences are important.

Abdul

Abdul was in his late 20s when he arrived in the UK, and this was the first time he had had to learn to use an English toilet. Prior to that he was used to using a toilet that did not involve sitting on a seat but rather squatting over a hole in the floor. Prior even to that, people would go into the fields in rural Pakistan to go to the toilet. A few years into his dementia, Abdul began passing his bowels while squatting over the navy-blue bath mat in the family bathroom. Unable to understand this behaviour, the family was convinced that his condition was deteriorating. They moved the navy-blue mat into one of the ensuite bathrooms and managed this change privately between themselves. Although this worked for six months, Abdul then began going into the garden to move his bowels. Worried for Abdul's dignity, the family called in the CPN to see if anything could be given to him to stop him from doing this. Tensions had risen in the house as family members used all efforts to stop this from happening.

Abdul had, of course, reverted to his time in Pakistan. First, the navy-blue mat was visually interpreted as a hole in the floor. If in a person's dementia, there is damage to the occipital lobe, this can quite often mean that two-dimensional and three-dimensional vision becomes affected. Just as a shiny floor can be interpreted as water, a dark-patched area can be seen as a step or a hole in the floor. Indeed, as the dementia progressed, his older memory became more prominent and Abdul reached a point where he was using the fields to pass urine and empty his bowels, which in the present day was the garden. A decision was made to create a safe private space for Abdul to do this, one where neighbours could not see him, and his dignity could be maintained.

The importance of understanding someone's life history was emphasised by Kitwood (1997), who highlighted that people with dementia must be cared for as individuals in the context of their unique identity and biography. Building on Kitwood's work, Brooker (2007) later developed the VIPS framework, which serves as a toolkit to support services to deliver care that: Values people, looks at Individual needs, understands the Perspective of the service user and provides a supportive Social psychology. Understanding the person's life history is crucial for delivering on any of these elements to provide high-quality care that is person centred.

As highlighted in the case examples, personal history-taking that considers the migration experiences of migrants is crucial for understanding behaviours and providing appropriate care. Such information should be documented on assessment and continued as an iterative process throughout treatment.

Working with South Asian communities: practice perspectives

In 1999, health and social care agencies in Wolverhampton (West Midlands) became aware of the large numbers of people from BAME communities and their under-representation in mental health services. Consequently, Fordementia (now Dementia UK) commissioned a research project that reviewed the relevant literature, engaged with local community leaders and organisations, and identified and interviewed people with suspected dementia and their carers from South Asian and African Caribbean communities (entitled Twice a Child I). The findings of this project in 2001 led to wide-ranging recommendations in several areas and a policy decision was made to appoint a CPN – an Asian link nurse (Harjinder Kaur) – to help implement these recommendations. As reported in Kaur *et al.* (2010), several activities were undertaken to reach out to the South Asian communities, including providing information via talks and presentations at local temples, mandirs and community centres. As the community began to come forth, diagnosis rates increased, and a carer support group was developed (Kaur *et al.* 2010).

Indeed, as highlighted by Blakemore *et al.* (2018), literacy issues in South Asian communities meant that reading and writing tests were not appropriate. Although several screening tools such as the Mini Mental State Examination (MMSE) and Addenbrooke's Cognitive Examination Version III (ACE III) are translated into Asian languages, cultural bias remains with use of these tools. Long-term memory testing may report false negatives due to differences in cultural, literacy and political issues in the person's country of origin. Blakemore *et al.* (2018), in their scoping review of the literature on dementia in UK South Asians, did not identify any studies that had addressed the introduction and validation of a purely diagnostic assessment for the UK South Asians, such as the ACE III or the Montreal Cognitive Assessment.

In her experience of diagnosing dementia in UK South Asian communities, and as a CPN, Harjinder Kaur reports challenges with differences in language, migration, culture, values and beliefs. The Rowland Universal Dementia Scale (RUDAS) is a relatively new tool in comparison with the MMSE and was developed in a multicultural setting in Australia. It is a brief six-item screening test that is short and easy to administer and, so far, is the most effective tool for diagnosing dementia in South Asian communities, according to Harjinder Kaur. It is effective because it relies in part on functional and practical tests. According to Harjinder Kaur, the tool is friendly and fun, takes away the fear of having an assessment done, the person does not have to admit that they cannot read or write, and the information from the initial assessment can be used to assist with the tool. You do, however, still need to be able to speak their language and dialects and ensure that they can hear you (and understand) and see you. There is still a need for validated culturally appropriate diagnostic tools for UK South Asians that can be applied on a much wider scale.

To develop an effective and appropriate care plan, assessments should involve several visits. This is even more important where assessments require a gender-sensitive approach. For example, Harjinder Kaur in her role as CPN found that a number of visits were required when assessing a male, as they tended not to disclose information immediately. Care plans require a multi-agency approach involving regular visits to evaluate the treatment put in place. It is also important that families are aware of the services available, particularly their financial entitlements, and, where possible, services such as day care and respite care should be promoted. One way to achieve this is to accompany the family to visit the prospective service.

Based on the feedback from education and training with healthcare professionals, language is seen as the biggest barrier for providing high-quality dementia care to UK South Asians. For example, Jutlla and Lillyman (2014) explored the challenges for healthcare professionals working with people with dementia from minority ethnic communities and found that the family were considered a key resource for helping the person with dementia to live well. A lack of communication and trust with family members not only resulted in limited information about the needs and wants of the person, but also caused staff to feel marginalised and excluded. Such feelings quite often led to a lack of motivation and self-worth for staff working with such people, particularly as it created an additional barrier for the staff caring for the person with dementia. The authors concluded that healthcare professionals, like most people, want to feel acknowledged and appreciated. This is a key area that needs addressing by creating innovative ways of improving communication and rapport between staff and family members. Despite this being an important area, we must not, however, forget that, first and foremost, staff are advocating care for the person with dementia and a reliance on family members for information can bring its own challenges. We must therefore ensure that staff are equipped with the skills and knowledge required to enable them to provide person-centred care that is also culturally competent. For Gallegos, Tindall and Gallegos (2008) cultural competence refers to:

> the process by which individuals and systems respond respectfully and effectively to people of all cultures, languages, classes, races, ethnic backgrounds, religions, and other diversity factors in a manner that recognises, affirms, and values the worth of individuals, families, and communities and protects and preserves the dignity of each.

It therefore involves more than having an awareness of cultural norms but rather represents a value-based perspective that recognises individuality. It also requires 'cultural humility', which is a lifelong commitment to self-evaluation and the awareness that one's own culture is not the only or best one (Schuessler, Wilder and Byrd 2012). As a concept, cultural competence deserves further research to take on board the lived experiences and ramifications of superdiversity in order to develop personalised nursing and care interventions based on known human needs and cultural diversity.

Summary

This chapter has discussed UK South Asians' understanding of dementia from a community perspective. It has highlighted the importance of migration and migrant identities for understanding the lived experience of dementia for such communities. We have drawn on our research and clinical expertise to explore these areas and provide practical guidance for individuals and organisations wanting to work with, and support, UK South Asian families living with dementia.

We recognise that the current evidence base regarding prevalence, diagnosis and service delivery in these communities is limited. Further research is required to develop culturally appropriate diagnostic tools and effective community engagement – which involves working collaboratively with community organisations, faith groups and families. This may involve creating innovative ways of improving communication and rapport between healthcare professionals and family members where language barriers exist.

As we move towards a more 'superdiverse' society, care must be personalised and tailored to meet individual and family needs. Furthermore, UK South Asians consist of many different communities who are by no means homogenous groups. As highlighted by the All Party Parliamentary Group on Dementia (2013, p.20):

[UK South Asians] share a similar experience and face particular challenges in getting the support they need. But nonetheless it is important to acknowledge and respond to the differences within ethnic groups and, at an individual level, ensure a person-centred approach is taken.

For this to be effective, we must promote and develop cultural competence as a set of congruent behaviours, knowledge, attitudes and policies that come together in a system, organisation or among professionals to enable effective work in cross-cultural situations (Lee and Farrell 2006).

References

All Party Parliamentary Group on Dementia (2013) *Dementia does not discriminate: The experiences of black, Asian and minority ethnic communities*. London: All Party Parliamentary Group on Dementia.

Blakemore, A., Kenning, C., Mirza, N., Daker-White, G., Panagioti, M. and Waheed, W. (2018). 'Dementia in UK South Asians: A scoping review of the literature.' *British Medical Journal*. doi:10.1136/bmjopen-2017-020290.

Brooker, D. (2007) *Person-Centred Dementia Care: Making Services Better*. London: Jessica Kingsley Publishers.

Department of Health (1998) *They Look After Their Own Don't They? Inspection of Community Care Services for Black and Minority Ethnic Older People*. London: Department of Health.

Differences Between (2018) *Differences Between Eastern and Western Philosophy*. Available at: www.differencebetween.net/science/differences-between-eastern-and-western-philosophy/#ixzz5R438a9tR [accessed 28/09/2018].

Gallegos, J.S., Tindall, C. and Gallegos, S.A. (2008) 'The need for advancement in the conteptualization of cultural competence.' *Advances in Social Work*, 9, 1, 51–62.

James, A.G. (1974) *Sikh Children in Britain*. London: Oxford University Press.

Jolley, D., Moreland, N., Read, K., Kaur, H., Jutlla, K. and Clark, M. (2009) 'The "Twice a Child" Projects: Learning about dementia and related disorders within the black and minority ethnic population of an English city and improving relevant services.' *Journal of Ethnicity and Inequalities in Health and Social Care*, 2, 4, 4–9.

Jutlla, K. (2011) *Caring for a Person with Dementia: A Qualitative Study of the Experiences of the Sikh Community in Wolverhampton*. British Library EThOS: Thesis, 356.

Jutlla, K. (2013) 'Ethnicity and cultural diversity in dementia care: A review of the research.' *Journal of Dementia Care*, 21, 2, 33–39.

Juttla K. (2014) 'The impact of migration experiences and migration identities on the experiences of services and caring for a family member with dementia for Sikhs living in Wolverhampton.' *UK Ageing and Society*/FirstView Article, July 2014, 1–23. doi: 10.1017/S0144686X14000658.

Jutlla, K. (2015) 'Dementia and Caregiving in South Asian Communities.' In J. Botsford and K. Harrison Denning *Dementia, Culture and Ethnicity: Issues for All*. London: Jessica Kingsley Publishers.

Jutlla, K. and Lillyman, S. (2014) 'An action research study engaging in the use of storyboarding as research-based teaching to identify issues faced when working with people with dementia from minority ethnic communities.' *Worcester Journal of Learning and Teaching*, 9, 23–35.

Jutlla, K. and Moreland, N. (2007) *Twice a Child III: The Experiences of Asian Carers of Older People with Dementia in Wolverhampton.* West Midlands: Fordementiaplus.

Jutlla, K. and Moreland, N. (2009) 'The personalisation of dementia services and existential realities: Understanding Sikh carers caring for an older person with dementia in Wolverhampton.' *Journal of Ethnicity and Inequalities in Health and Social Care,* 2, 4, 10–21.

Kaur, H., Jutlla, K., Moreland, N. and Read, K. (2010) 'How a link nurse ensured equal treatment for people of Asian origin with dementia.' *Nursing Times,* 106, 24, 4–9.

Kenning, C., Daker-White, G., Blakemore, A., Panagioti, M. and Waheed, W. (2017) 'Barriers and facilitators in accessing dementia care by ethnic minority groups: A meta-synthesis of qualitative studies.' *BMC Psychiatry,* 17, 316.

Kitwood, T. (1997) *Dementia Reconsidered: The Person Comes First.* Buckingham: Open University Press.

Lee, S.A. and Farrell, M. (2006) 'Is cultural competency a backdoor to racism?' *Rethinking Race and Human Variation* special edition. American Anthropological Association.

Mackenzie, J. (2007) 'Ethnic Minority Communities and the Experience of Dementia: A Review and Implications for Practice.' In J. Keady, L.C. Clarke and S. Page *Partnerships in Community Mental Health Nursing and Dementia Care: Practice Perspectives.* Maidenhead: Open University Press.

Moriarty, J., Sharif, N. and Robinson, J. (March 2011) *Black and minority ethnic people with dementia and their access to support and services.* Research Briefing. Social Care Institute for Excellence.

Regan, J.L. (2014) 'Redefining dementia care barriers for ethnic minorities: The religion-culture distinction.' *Journal of Mental Health, Religion & Culture.* 17, 4, 345–353.

Schuessler, J.B. Wilder, B. and Byrd, L.W. (2012) 'Reflective journaling and development of cultural humility in students.' *Nursing Education Perspectives,* 33, 2, 96–99.

Seabrooke, V. and A. Milne (Jan 2004) *Culture and Care in Dementia: A Study of the Asian Community in Northwest Kent, UK.* London: Mental Health Foundation.

CHAPTER 5

Dementia and the UK Chinese Community

David Truswell, Tom Lam and Gill Tan

Historical connections between China and the UK

The many trading routes between Europe and China that became latterly
known as the Silk Road have existed since the time of the Roman Empire
and it has been argued the Chinese technological innovations of printing,
the compass, and gunpowder were critical for the emergence of the European
Renaissance (Shaffer 1986). A significant step in reinforcing the global
economic power of the British Empire in the 18th century was the East India
Company becoming the leading supplier of opium to the Chinese market
in 1773. Britain at the time had a monopoly on the production of opium in
colonial Bengal and this was sold to purchase Chinese products such as silks
then in high demand in the British and European markets. At the time, the
sale and smoking of opium in China was prohibited by Chinese imperial
decree. The scale of the UK trade in illegal opium was subsequently to lead
two Opium Wars (1839–42) and (1856–60) (*Encyclopedia Britannica*, n.d.).

The long-standing nature of the historical, cultural and economic contact
between China and the UK is rarely acknowledged in mainstream UK
historical narratives; the Chinese contribution to UK history and culture is
often confined to a narrow stereotype of Chinese restaurants and takeaways
and Kung-Fu movies. Yet, Chinese migrants to the UK made an important
contribution to the war effort in World War II. In 1939, the Chinese
Merchant Seaman's Pool established in Liverpool had 20,000 members.
The UK post-war reconstruction period saw a substantial increase in ethnic
Chinese migration to the UK, from Malaysia, Hong Kong and Guangdong
province in China.

Economic push-and-pull factors over the generations have had an impact on the type of ethnic Chinese migrating to the UK, reflected in the variety of countries of origin of those who are ethnically Chinese and the variety in basic education level and pre-existing familiarity of the Chinese migrants with the English language over the years. The contemporary UK Chinese migrant population, in common with many UK settled migrant populations, is heterogenous and often has a lifetime experience of racial discrimination in the UK. It also has a generationally differentiated experience of migration, globally dispersed family relationships, and the experience of cultural discontinuity when facing the challenge of adapting to new cultural expectations through migration. Migrants who regard themselves as ethnically Chinese may originate from a variety of national backgrounds apart from mainland China, including Malaysia, Vietnam, Taiwan, Hong Kong (only recently politically reunited with China) and a variety of other countries with long-standing Chinese populations. Within China itself it is estimated that 90 per cent of Chinese citizens classify themselves as ethnically Han Chinese but there are also other ethnic Chinese identities.

Dementia research and the Chinese community in the UK

The political and social circumstances of UK Black, Asian and minority ethnic (BAME) communities often leads to mainstream health research narratives viewing migrant populations as an ethnic population segment detached from the population in the country of origin. In the 21st century, this may be too limiting when attempting to understand the family social dynamic impact of dementia and issues such as the economic impact of dementia on transnational family networks. The ethnic Chinese world encompasses both some of the most sophisticated of modern healthcare and some of the world's most impoverished regions. Intergenerational changes in healthcare expectations and the ability to make international comparisons in care provision, anecdotally at least, can feature in the accounts of family carers from the Chinese community where some aspects of dementia services in developed areas of the Chinese world (for example, Hong Kong) may be regarded as superior to those in the UK (Bristol BME People Dementia Research Group 2017).

A 2017 World Health Organization report (Xu *et al.* 2017) points out that China has the largest population of people living with dementia, rising from an estimated 44.4 million in 2013 to an estimated 75.6 million by 2030. This is across a rapidly growing elderly population in a country that is also rapidly industrialising and becoming a major international economic force with massive population shifts from rural living to urbanisation and modernisation. However, a systematic review by Lang *et al.* (2017) indicates that China has some of the poorest rates of dementia detection in the world, particularly for those Chinese people with low economic status. Work by Chen *et al.* (2013) has indicated under-diagnosis of dementia and depression in later life in rural China of over 90 per cent. Historic events, such as the one-child policy on the mainland and the strong cultural imperative for family-based support, have important repercussions for dementia care across the Chinese world, including migrant Chinese communities.

Stereotypical notions of Chinese filial care fail to take account of the impact of a generation of mainly single children or take account of observations such as those of Chen *et al.* (2014) that the cultural norm in rural China is to regard people living with dementia as 'crazy' and often respond to them with ridicule, isolation and abuse. A further blow to the stereotypical assumption of filial care in the UK Chinese community is dealt by the work of Li *et al.* (1999) who, when looking at the mental health needs of the UK Chinese communities, found that Chinese people in the UK living with mental health issues often experienced loneliness, social exclusion and harassment from the Chinese community. Chinese families in the UK may be more isolated than other migrant communities through geographical dispersion across the UK and are also less likely to form social networks through faith communities. At the same time, children may fear being portrayed as heartless if they think of moving a parent living with dementia into a care home when struggling with other family support and work pressures (All Party Parliamentary Group on Dementia 2013).

There is little research done on the impact of dementia in the UK Chinese community. The lack of information in this area and the stigma surrounding mental health issues often leave Chinese people living with dementia, and their family carers, in an isolated position within their communities, as well as receiving a poor response from mainstream support services.

The experience of dementia in the UK Chinese community

While the Chinese written language is commonly shared by ethnic Chinese, there is no single spoken Chinese language. As well as the more well-known Chinese languages, Cantonese and Mandarin, many ethnic Chinese may speak other language variants, such as Hakka, which are more common in specific regions of China or other countries of origin for ethnic Chinese. Migrants with limited or no education may not have spoken much English, despite having lived for many years in the UK, as they have lived entirely within the UK Chinese environment, possibly working in the catering and restaurant trades. Chinese people who do not have English as a first language may lose their English language skills as their dementia progresses. The Chinese language terms for dementia are usually derogatory terms with some sense of meaning 'mad' or 'crazy' (Chen *et al.* 2014). The association of dementia with mental illness means dementia can attract the stigma associated with mental illness in the Chinese community, leading the family to fear social isolation and to isolate the person living with dementia from contact with the community or to marginalise or try to minimise the problem by explaining it as an inevitable consequence of ageing. Cultural social norms such as 'keeping face' lead people to avoid acknowledging problems or looking for help, keeping up an appearance of coping or avoiding exposing themselves to possible social shame.

Some older Chinese first-generation migrants in the UK may have remained in close contact with their Chinese cultural heritage to the point of continuing to read Chinese newspapers or largely consume Chinese language media for most of their lives, even while encouraging their UK-born offspring to integrate with UK culture and speak English as the route to educational achievement and career progress in the UK. This may leave children, for example, unable to find common ground to communicate with parents who develop dementia. As English-speaking and educated offspring, they are faced with communicating with a parent or grandparent who has reverted to an exclusive use of language they were discouraged from using (Truswell *et al.* 2015) and cultural materials they may be unfamiliar with. Clinical services may have little experience in working with people from the Chinese community and may not know where to source appropriate community intelligence and resources in that community.

The Chinese community in the UK is relatively dispersed, and healthcare and social support are strongly associated with family bonds and cultural traditions of family obligation between family members that emphasise the filial duties of children towards parents. However, contemporary circumstances and the impact of migration have important consequences for family support systems that call into question any assumption by services that families will characteristically 'look after their own'. Culturally, dementia has been a stigmatised disease, and for families that are transnationally dispersed because of migration there may be no family members physically close enough to provide the continuing personal oversight and support needed as dementia progresses. Also, first-generation migrants may either not marry or have children or may have partners from other cultures, and their children may not have the same set of cultural expectations.

While the Chinese community in the UK is very dispersed compared with other minority ethnic communities, there are some significant metropolitan locations that provide an important cultural and social focus. London's Chinatown may be the best known in the UK, but 'Chinatown' areas exist in Manchester, Birmingham, Liverpool and Newcastle and have done for some time. Chinese voluntary organisations exist at a local level; for example, there are several borough-based Chinese organisations in London, and also Chinese organisations and associations that function at a regional or national level. In London, there are Chinese voluntary organisations that have strong local connections but serve a particular purpose that gives them both a strong London-wide and also national role – for example, the Chinese National Healthy Living Centre based in Soho and the Chinese Mental Health Association who have services in a number of London boroughs. As well as Chinese health and care organisations, there are also Chinese business networks that exist at regional and national levels.

Chinese UK voluntary organisations often have excellent proactive networking, both with other Chinese organisations and with other non-Chinese agencies, and are a significant social and information resource for UK Chinese migrants. They undoubtably provide an anchoring point for personal and community resilience for the UK Chinese community but often are either unknown to or ignored by mainstream health and care services as a potential partner in providing health information to the Chinese community and the delivery of health and care services. As an example, recent efforts by the Chinese National Healthy Living Centre to get national-level data on the use of dementia services from mainstream providers of dementia services in both the statutory and voluntary sector were largely unsuccessful due to the lack of recording of Chinese ethnicity by most of the organisations approached. Ethnicity data on dementia for a study in Bristol (Bristol BME People Dementia Research Group 2017) indicates a significant under-representation when comparing the numbers of people of Chinese ethnicity accessing services with the census-based projection of the local number of Chinese people living with dementia.

Stigma regarding dementia, feelings of obligation to provide family care for elderly parents and the experience of discrimination or fear of experiencing discrimination from services all contribute to a reluctance of Chinese people in the UK to engage not only with dementia services but many health services. One comes across clinicians and researchers who assume a degree of vigour, resilience and good health in the Chinese population. These clinicians and researchers seen unaware of some of the substantial health and social issues of concern for the UK Chinese community, examples of this being smoking and gambling. This is often accompanied by a presumption by health professionals of the Chinese community 'looking after its own', with scant evidence to confirm the truth or falsity of this assertion.

May's story

May (not her real name) is Chinese, a retired community mental health nurse and a full-time carer for her English husband who is living with dementia. She has no paid carers supporting her and does not claim any care allowance. She has been going to a monthly group for Chinese carers of people living with dementia that was supported by the Chinese National Healthy Living Centre's Dementia Project and she also goes to a support group in Greenwich. She enjoys the Chinese carers' group and has involved herself and her husband and two other Chinese couples. The group has a warm-up with physical exercise and Gill, the Chinese dementia support worker, has arranged talks, for example on lasting power of attorney. It is a good place to share experiences, with a lot of comparisons to talk about.

She and her husband also regularly attend a support group in Greenwich, which May is really pleased with because it has more volunteer workers and they can give more time for individual support. They have done things like structured reminiscence sessions looking at life development in a step-by-step way, concentrating on people's memories from different stages in their lives. One of the reminiscence sessions on sports was particularly useful as May's husband used to be a sports coach in schools. The volunteer had pictures illustrating different sports and was able to help him express more through using the pictures. If the reminiscence had only been verbal, he wouldn't have been able to express himself so much.

Day-to-day communication with her husband has become difficult; for example, they were recently sitting at home and watching two men in the road outside who were trying to repair their car that was parked across the way from the house. Her husband was convinced they were up to no good and kept insisting May needed to do something about them.

As May is retired, she wants to continue to ensure that her husband is still involved in activities that make life enjoyable, but this can be a struggle. She recently took him along for a 'Singing for the Brain' session but she could see he wasn't really enjoying it. He kept forgetting the words of the song. He had lost the words, so he couldn't sing. They tried to get him more involved by giving him a tambourine, but he quickly put it down.

Something like a Christmas party or festive party he can still enjoy. He was a good dancer and he has enjoyed himself when he has had the chance to dance with some ladies at an event. But now, some of the old ladies do not want to dance with him because they can't raise their arms and can't do the dances anymore. They refuse to dance with him when he asks them, and May thinks he does not understand why they are refusing.

One of the most difficult aspects of daily life that has changed is that he no longer shares the housework. May might want him to take a bag of rubbish out to the wheelie bin but he does not understand where or what the wheelie bin is. Other things he does not understand are daily objects - if she asks him to get her a knife, he will give her a comb instead. He does not understand the differences between the men and women's toilet signs, so May prefers to take him or go inside with him to the disabled toilet because he forgets to wash his hands after using the toilet in their house. Once when she took him shopping in the supermarket, while she was looking at the price and the quality of an article, a shop assistant came and told her, 'Your husband just used one of our buckets to pass urine.' May was so embarrassed and apologised to them, explaining that he had dementia. Fortunately, they were understanding. Now, every time they go shopping she feels she has to watch him like a hawk in case any unpleasant incident happens. The routines of everyday life feel like an up-hill struggle. She feels she can't expect any help from him at all and says he can't even make a cup of tea for himself. He is still continent and can feed and dress himself without assistance, but May has to help him with bathing. At night, he has a bucket near his bedside, so that he can use it to pass urine three or four times a night.

As her husband is English, May thinks there may be some differences between what she sees as her role as a carer in their 'mixed marriage' and the situation for a Chinese couple. But what Chinese people think they should do is not always the same for all Chinese people. She met a Chinese couple on one occasion and when she asked the wife if she was worried about her husband who is living with dementia getting lost, the wife's response was basically 'if he gets lost, he gets lost'. This surprised May, and the lady went on to explain that her husband had wandered off several times in the past and she expected him to be found eventually by someone and reported.

May didn't understand this at all. Her husband had recently left on his own when she thought he was going to wait for her while she finished getting prepared to leave the house. She went to look for him but had no idea where he was. She was nearly panicked and close to crying. Fortunately, she was rung by the local pharmacist who had found her husband and said that he was clearly in a confused state. She could never take the attitude 'if he gets lost, he gets lost'.

The story of Gileng and her grandmother

Gileng is married with two children and combines being a mother with running a private catering business in Hertfordshire. Her sister has three children and lives in West London. They have both always been close to their grandmother (Mrs C), a fiercely independent Chinese lady from Malaysia who was widowed at the age of 19 and raised Gileng's father as a single parent. Mrs C had been working as a bursar in a prestigious school in Malaysia but she followed her son to London in the 1960s to help in the family restaurant business and with childcare for Gileng and her sister. She then worked as an NHS cleaner at the Whittington Hospital, London, for about 20 years, initially living in nurses' accommodation attached to the hospital.

Gileng is now estranged from her father, and her mother and father separated when Gileng and her sister were very young. Mrs C played a significant role in looking after Gileng and her sister as they grew up. Mrs C was always a self-reliant and socially active woman. She was one of the founder members of the Islington Chinese Association and volunteered as a cook providing lunches for the Chinese community as well as attending a variety of activities, including fan dancing and calligraphy. She moved into her own flat in the North London area and continued to keep in regular contact with Gileng and her sister as they got older, cooking a meal and inviting them over to the flat on a regular basis.

The first major sign that something had changed for Mrs C was about nine years ago when Gileng arrived at a familiar meeting point in West London to pick her up and take her to a niece's tenth birthday party, only to find she was nowhere to be seen. The birthday was a big family occasion that had been planned for some time, but when Gileng went round to Mrs C's flat searching for her she found Mrs C at home with no idea about the big occasion. There had been a few times over the previous months when her grandmother had what seemed to be mini-strokes and she had at one point developed Bell's palsy, but this seemed much more serious.

In fact, it was the start of a more consistent and marked period of decline in Mrs C's health. Her fastidious care of her flat and her personal appearance began to wane. She would remove food from the freezer and leave it in the sink for days on end. She began to neglect her own personal care. A phone call from the police was received after she was found wandering and confused in the Swiss Cottage area of London at 4am.

Gileng and her sister tried to support her as much as they could but they lived outside London and also had to balance other family and work demands. They were given help and advice by dementia support workers from the local Chinese community organisation and by local social services. The community organisation provided a regular lunch club. It was the lunch club volunteer who went round to Mrs C's house when she failed to turn up for the lunch club and found her looking pale and clammy. The volunteer took her to the hospital and she was found to have broken her arm and badly bruised her hip in a fall. The volunteer contacted Gileng's sister to let her know. Over the next few days, Mrs C made constant calls to both Gileng and her sister as she was in pain from her hip and arm but did not know why. The arm fracture was awkwardly located and she was treated by placing the arm in a sling instead of having it plastered. Gileng and her sister would visit to find she had removed the sling because she had forgotten why it was in place.

Despite keeping Mrs C at home with regular visits, home carer support and digital independent living aids, the situation continued to deteriorate. Mrs C failed to recognise the home carers, she forgot to wear alert pendants, she dismantled alarm monitors for fire and gas detection and was completely disoriented by remote call systems that for her were just mysterious voices from nowhere. There were more occasions when Mrs C would be found wandering at night, and concern for her safety was increasing.

An initial attempt at finding a suitable care home in Mrs C's local borough was unsuccessful but now she is living in a small home local to Gileng with a Cantonese-speaking manager from Singapore. About 50 per cent of the other residents are Chinese. While Gileng and her sister have some ability to converse in Cantonese, they have been concerned about their ability to be the best interpreters for their grandmother in the clinical settings. Their grandmother converses now entirely in her mother tongue. Mrs C seems happy and settled in her new home and Gileng and her sister take her out for a meal in a local restaurant every month. Mrs C still also has contact with her great-grandchildren who appreciate that she is living with dementia. A constantly difficult part of the monthly meal, however, is that Mrs C will become very anxious and sometimes quite distressed as the meal draws to a close and want to have access to her handbag and her keys to go 'home'. This is usually resolved once she is back inside the care home as she has positive feelings about the home and she does not make any references to her previous London flat.

Gileng feels that the support of the local Chinese community organisation and the lunch club service in London area where her grandmother lived were exemplary as was that of the local social services staff. Getting early advice about setting up lasting power of attorney for Mrs C's financial affairs was particularly important for arranging subsequent care and dealing with ongoing payments on her behalf.

A dilemma Gileng and her sister struggled with for a long time was how much to get involved in organising help for Mrs C and balance this with respecting their grandmother's lifelong spirited independence, particularly how they could do this without Mrs C feeling threatened with losing 'face'. Gileng describes 'face' as the idea that Chinese people must always say everything is alright and not talk about having problems. This is obviously a cultural attribute that serves a new migrant well in being resilient to the obstacles of making a new life in an unfamiliar country but can inhibit both looking for and using help in the circumstances of developing dementia. It also will continue to be an ongoing personal and family concern of someone who is Chinese living with dementia.

The Chinese National Healthy Living Centre Dementia Project

The Chinese National Healthy Living Centre (CNHLC) received funding from London's City Bridge Fund for a dementia support and awareness-raising project that started in January 2014 with the following objectives:

- To remove or reduce stigma attached to dementia among the Chinese community.
- To raise awareness about dementia (symptoms, prevention, treatment) among Chinese people.
- To give support to people living with dementia, and their carers (through advice, home visits and training).
- To promote a positive attitude about dementia and encourage service users to test/take prevention measures (e.g. changing eating habits, stop smoking).

The work had a London-wide remit and over the past five years has worked with 13 other Chinese community group organisations, holding awareness workshops both at its own premises and those of these groups. These workshops have included speakers on a variety of aspects of dementia from a number of organisations, including the Alzheimer's Society, Greenwich Memory Clinic, One Westminster, Right at Home, Home Instead, Kingston University, Westminster Dementia Advice, Tzu Chi Foundation, Westminster Admiral Nurses and several others. Over 40 volunteers have been recruited and trained by the project over its lifetime; some for the short term, others for nearly three years. The key full-time paid role of dementia support worker in the project has been split between two bilingual post-holders who have been with the project since its inception. The project has reached 1000 Chinese people a year, achieving a total of 5000 by the time the project funding finished at the end of 2018.

Initially, the project's target was to reach out to around 1000 people each year through workshops, carers' group meetings (tea houses), home visits, publicity materials (leaflets, newspaper bulletins, and TV/radio announcements). It worked with London Spectrum International (a community language station based in London) to publicise and promote services and activities. Two dementia booklets and several leaflets were produced by translating the English originals from professional bodies, and copies of these were widely distributed across London. Until 2016, when the London-based Chinese TV channel ceased to broadcast, its audience included Chinese listeners in 24 countries in the European continent. The project has also translated into Chinese several booklets about dementia for other organisations.

A national conference on dementia in the Chinese community was organised in 2016 at China Exchange (Chinatown, London), attended by nearly 170 delegates. The conference was video linked to another Chinese community audience of over 90 in Newcastle. The conference attracted quite a few community leaders, specialists in the field, and some well-known faces as well as members of the public.

Of those who attended the workshops and the various activities and meetings, 65 per cent referred themselves after being informed by the project's publicity (radio, newspaper bulletins), 10 per cent were referred to the project by other organisations/surgeries, and another 25 per cent by other community organisations.

The project developed a new Chinese term for dementia. The existing Chinese term was translated in such a way that a person living with dementia could be seen as foolish, crazy, and slow in thinking and responding. The new Chinese term 'tui-zhi-zheng' is used for CNHLC's website and has been adopted widely within the UK's Chinese community (Chinese TV/radio/newspapers). Some health professionals visiting from the Far East have also commented positively on this new translation. A senior lecturer from University College London's translation department is now working with the project to produce an app of dementia terms in Chinese, and 'tui-zhi-zheng' is the terms used for this.

The work of the project was led by two bilingual Chinese dementia support workers who job-shared a full-time post and who are contributing co-authors of this chapter (Tom Lam and Gill Tan). Discussion of their experience as dementia support workers yielded the following observations:

- The Chinese community in the UK is diverse: language/dialect/regional backgrounds need different approaches for different individuals (e.g. use of dialects, advice on regional customs/eating preferences).
- Many contemporary older Chinese people in the UK have worked in labour-intensive sectors, such as restaurants/takeaways (where the kitchen in many cases is in the basement). The phrase 'a life in the dark' is a common expression used by kitchen workers referring to the downside of their occupation (it's dark in the basement when they are working, and when finishing work in the evening, the sky is dark again, especially in winter). They say that this is the reason for them not having time to attend English classes and socialise.
- Limited language skills, coupled with cultural barriers, cause more problems for Chinese elders if they are housed in a residential home.
- Older Chinese people have a different perception of being healthy. For many, being healthy is just 'having no illness', rather than being mentally and physically energetic and active. Some therefore shy away from accessing healthcare services for what they think are 'minor problems'.
- Language barriers between older people and their western-educated children can create communication difficulties. In one case, the GP son of a patient could not explain things in the mother tongue to his parent.

- Lack of English puts older Chinese people in a vulnerable situation when it comes to using equipment with English-only instructions, such as dementia trackers and computer software for memory tests. It can also hamper their ability to claim the benefits they are entitled to.

- Traditional Chinese family values are changing. Young people prefer to move out instead of living with their parents, not only in the UK and Europe but also in mainland China. Rapid economic development and financial gain have allowed many young people in China to move into cities, leaving their parents behind in the countryside where the living conditions remain far from desirable. Instead of looking after their elderly parents as before, successful young people can now hire carers to handle the care.

- Older generations of Chinese (in fact, even some younger people) place considerable weight on Chinese traditional medicine for certain illnesses and many spend large sums of their income and savings on private treatment, like acupuncture. A person finding themselves forgetful may insist on visiting a Chinese drug shop to buy Chinese herbs rather than having a memory test.

- Many people living with dementia, and in many cases their family members, are reluctant to admit having the problem. The CNHLC Project has identified a number of Chinese people living with dementia, either with onset symptoms or with more advanced illness, but only about one-third were willing to receive befrienders. Some took no further visits after the first fact-finding one.

Through the project, understanding about dementia among the Chinese population has improved. Following the five years' work across the London boroughs involved, there are few people who are members of the community centres that the project worked with who have not been informed of the disease in some way. Carers who took part in the tea house meetings and training sessions have gained even more understanding about the people they are looking after.

The project has also helped to raise CNHLC's profile within the community care sector, through partnership and mutual support with other community organisations and NHS healthcare providers. At this point in time, the CNHLC has run one of the largest dementia awareness projects for the Chinese community in the UK. The project has also allowed CNHLC to be seen as a stronghold for translating dementia-related literature into Chinese languages.

The project has involved a multi-method approach to raising awareness in a population with poor engagement with mainstream dementia services and considerable cultural stigma regarding dementia. A culturally appropriate information and support approach grew out of the workshops and was dubbed the 'reminiscence tea house', developing a distinctive Chinese remodelling of the well-known 'dementia cafe' model. The 'tea house' includes people living with dementia, and their carers, and the project delivered a programme of information sessions through the 'tea house', including invited speakers. Each local 'tea house' developed its own programme of sessions and invited speakers following discussions with the 'tea house' members.

Supporting people in the Chinese community living with dementia

The historical connection between the Chinese community and the UK is more long-standing than is often appreciated in the UK mainstream. As China continues to grow in dominance in the global economy, financial investment in the UK and the value the Chinese place on the UK university system as an education destination for its young people will continue to increase China's significance for the UK economy. Mainstream services in the UK largely misconceive the Chinese community as homogenous and generously supplied with family carers, and assume a level of general health in the UK older Chinese population for which there is no objective basis. For the CNHLC Dementia Project, an attempt to seek national-level data on the numbers of Chinese people in NHS older people's services, or using the services of major national older people's services and dementia charities, was unsuccessful because there was insufficient ethnicity recording (Eddie Chan, Chief Executive Officer of CNHLC, personal communication, 2018). The professional assumption seems to be that when Chinese people are not appearing in primary care statistics and memory service data, this reflects as them being less likely to get dementia. The work of CNHLC indicates that a more likely explanation is that Chinese people living with dementia, and their carers, are simply less likely to seek services. The creative approach of the CNHLC Dementia Project and the nuanced picture of the contemporary UK Chinese community that arises illustrate the value of a focused approach to dementia awareness-raising for this community. This is an illustration of the kind of targeted information campaign advocated by the All Party Parliamentary Group on Dementia report *Dementia does not discriminate* (2013).

The CNHLC Dementia Project demonstrates the capacity of the voluntary sector to organise and deliver a complex and multi-partnered health education and carer support initiative that also forges community links and supports resilience-building within the community. Health and social care commissioners need much more actively to seek out and support these initiatives with much clearer leadership from policy in this area than currently exists. Chinese people living with dementia face additional struggles with cultural stigma and 'loss of face' in seeking help for dementia, whether from professional services or within their own family and community. While these cultural barriers can be mitigated by funding work such as that provided by the CNHLC Dementia Project, a further important cultural barrier is the professionals' stereotyping of the Chinese person living with dementia, and their support network. Professional services need to reach out to Chinese community organisations proactively and with much more respect and humility to secure help with breaking down these cultural stereotypes and creating a more appropriate and inclusive dementia pathway for Chinese people.

References

All Party Parliamentary Group on Dementia (2013) *Dementia does not discriminate: The experiences of black, Asian and minority ethnic communities.* London: All Party Parliamentary Group on Dementia.

Bristol BME People Dementia Research Group (2017) *The Dementia Experiences of People from Caribbean, Chinese and South Asian Communities in Bristol.* Available at: www.bristolhealthpartners.org.uk/uploads/documents/2017-02-23/1487859789-dementia-needs-of-people-from-bme-communities-in-bristol.pdf [accessed 17/10/2018].

Chen, R., Hu, Z., Chen, R., Ma, Y., Zhang, D. and Wilson, K. (2013) 'Determinants for undetected dementia and late-life depression.' *British Journal of Psychiatry*, 203, 3, 203–208. doi:10.1192/bjp.bp.112.119354.

Chen, S., Boyle, L., Conwell, Y., Xiao, S. and Fung Kum Chiu, H. (2014) 'The challenges of dementia care in rural China.' *International Psychogeriatrics*, 26(7): 1059–1064. doi:10.1017/S1041610214000854.

Encyclopedia Britannica (n.d.) *The Opium Trade – British and Chinese History.* Available at: www.britannica.com/topic/opium-trade [accessed 15/10/2018].

Lang, L., Clifford, A., Wei, L., Zhang, D. *et al.* (2017) 'Prevalence and determinants of undetected dementia in the community: a systematic literature review and a meta-analysis.' *BMJ Open*, 7: e011146. doi: 10.1136/bmjopen-2016-011146 [accessed 17/10/2018].

Li, P-L., Logan, S., Yee, L. and Ng, S. (1999) 'Barriers to meeting the mental health needs of the Chinese community.' *Journal of Public Health Medicine*, 21, 1, 74–80.

Shaffer, L. (1986) *China, Technology and Change.* World History Bulletin, Fall/Winter World History Association. Available at: http://afe.easia.columbia.edu/chinawh/web/help/readings.html [accessed 15/10/2018].

Truswell, D., Leung, M., Lam, T. and Tan, G. (2015) 'The reminiscence tea house.' *Journal of Dementia Care*, 23, 3, 12–14.

Xu, J., Wang, J., Wimo, A., Fratiglioni, L. and Qiu, C. (2017) 'The economic burden of dementia in China, 1990–2030: Implications for health policy.' *Bulletin of the World Health Organization*, 95, 18–26. Available at: http://dx.doi.org/10.2471/BLT.15.167726 [accessed 17/10/2018].

CHAPTER 6

Supporting People Living with Dementia in the Jewish Community

Padraic Garrett

Older Jewish people in the UK living with dementia

There are approximately 270,000 Jews living in the UK. There are numerous Jewish charities working with older people and people living with dementia, including Jewish Care, Nightingale Hammerson, and Edinburgh House in London and the South East, Birmingham Jewish Community Care, and The Fed in Manchester, and Leeds Jewish Welfare Board. This chapter outlines the approach and experience of Jewish Care in supporting people living with dementia. Jewish Care is a leading communal organisation. It is the largest health and social care charity for the Jewish community in the UK, touching the lives of 10,000 people every week with a wide range of services from youth clubs to residential nursing homes. The organisation employs 1300 staff from multi-cultural backgrounds, together with 3000 volunteers who help maintain our services.

Based on statistics from the 2011 census, the Jewish population has a slightly higher median age than the general population, being 41 years compared with 39 years. Proportionately, there are significantly more people over 80 and over 85 than in the general population. In 2011, 21 per cent of the Jewish population in the UK were over 65. Given that statistically the prevalence of dementia is greater as age advances, and particularly for people over 80, clearly the Jewish community has a significant challenge to meet.

Jewish Care – working with dementia in the Jewish community

As in most communities, the Jewish community's understanding and awareness of dementia has grown significantly over the past 20 years. Jewish Care embraced the shift in thinking on dementia care from a medicalised model where people with dementia were treated as patients to a model where their social, cognitive and psychological wellbeing is highlighted. It adopted what Kitwood (1997) described as the person-centred approach. This is an approach that focuses on authentic contact and communication. Kitwood described person-centred care as ways of working that emphasise communication and relationships. This way of working with and understanding people living with dementia has developed into the relationship-centred approach. The relationship-centred approach recognises the importance of building and strengthening relationships and that this remains very important for people living with dementia.

As a community organisation, Jewish Care finds that the relationship-centred approach fits perfectly with the idea of belonging to the Jewish community and maintaining this identity. Jewish Care is guided by the principles of the organisation My Home Life[1] and its relationship-centred care, and the six senses framework developed by Mike Nolan and a team at Sheffield University (Nolan *et al.* 2006). They identify three groups of people in care settings: older people, families and staff. Jewish Care promotes a culture where these groups work together in keeping with its ethos as a community organisation that is striving to promote community. The six senses framework promotes the view that older people, relatives and staff all need to feel a sense of:

- security (to feel safe)
- continuity (to experience links and connections)
- belonging (to feel part of things)
- purpose (to have a goal to aspire to)
- fulfilment (to make progress towards these goals)
- significance (to feel that you matter as a person).

In 2009, the government launched *Living Well with Dementia: A National Strategy* (Department of Health 2009) in which it outlined a comprehensive range of initiatives to support people living with dementia from early stages

---

1   http://myhomelife.org.uk/good-practice/relationship-centred-care

of end of life. Jewish Care took the ethos of this strategy to develop its own dementia strategy. The implementation of its organisational strategy for dementia care was contained within a framework containing the three main aims of the national strategy. Below a summary of the strategy is outlined, together with the progress made.

Dementia and the strategic aims of Jewish Care

Strategic aim 1: To raise a better understanding of dementia in the Jewish community and address any misconceptions about the condition

There was a general understanding of dementia within the Jewish community, as in the wider community, but it was badly informed and many people regarded it as an inevitable part of ageing. The Jewish community, like the wider community, tended towards a view that there was little or nothing that could be done for people living with dementia. There often was a stigma associated with dementia, and a reluctance to talk about it. This could result in people with dementia becoming isolated and withdrawing from active membership in the community and this was often true for their partners and family carers too. The status quo was not to talk about dementia and sometimes that was because of being frightened about it.

For the past 12 years, Jewish Care has worked with the local Jewish community through networks, engaging with synagogues and schools to promote a better understanding of dementia. Since 2012, Jewish Care has run Dementia Friends programmes with Dementia Friends Champions. It has also promoted the idea of the Jewish community becoming a dementia-friendly community. The awareness and understanding of dementia has grown significantly and synagogues' social welfare workers are shifting ways to working with people living with dementia to more person-centred and relationship-centred approaches. This is ongoing work and requests for training and support come in regularly to Jewish Care from synagogues and other community groups.

A series of informative articles on dementia were run in the Jewish newspapers. The message that has been promoted is that people can live well with dementia with the right care and support. Supporting people with dementia to retain their links with the community has been a primary message, along with emphasising the importance of families and other communal networks welcoming them and adapting to their changing needs. The Jewish community has also benefited from the national dementia awareness programmes run by the Alzheimer's Society and a more positive and informative approach towards dementia in the media. Jewish Care has also worked to promote an attitude within the community to face the challenges of dementia together. The work of Jewish Care and other welfare groups within the community has seen a gradual change from being afraid to talk about dementia to being more open and working together to face the challenge. It has also been cognisant of pointing out the value that people living with dementia continue to bring to the community. Awareness-raising of the role, importance and experiences of family carers of people living with dementia has been equally vital. It has been significant to see schools reaching into care homes and day centres and giving their students opportunities to learn about dementia and, more importantly, to mix with people living with dementia from an early age.

The high number of community members volunteering in Jewish Care's services has been a very important aspect of promoting positive messages about dementia. When volunteers come forward, they receive training and information. They have opportunities to see how to work to improve the lives of people living with dementia and to see the possibilities for living well with the condition. The volunteers often become the advocates and champions in their communities, reducing stigma and demonstrating ways of making a difference for people with dementia and their families. Volunteering is often a way that family carers choose to continue to work in the community after the person they have been caring for has died. They choose to contribute the skills and knowledge they have learned through their family caring role to improve the lives of other people living with dementia. Volunteering can be a great source of fulfilment for them and a way of giving back to a community that has cared and been supportive.

Strategic aim 2: Ensuring that members of the Jewish community receive early diagnosis of dementia and access to support services

Jewish Care's strategic implementation in this area has concentrated on ensuring that people living with dementia, and their family carers, have access to effective services for early diagnosis and are guided to the most appropriate support from this point onwards. Early diagnosis empowers people to participate in planning their own future. The Jewish community is largely proactive in seeking advice and diagnoses for health-related issues. However, there tends to be a view that a diagnosis of dementia is of little help because there is no cure. Jewish Care has worked to promote an awareness that support, advice, services and treatments are available and that they can make a great difference to the wellbeing of the person living with dementia, and their family carer.

Jewish Care has a comprehensive pathway of support for people living with dementia, and their carers. Typically, the first point of contact is the Jewish Care Helpline, which is a free service. Helpline staff are trained to work with people with dementia and are knowledgeable about services available locally. The helpline team will either refer a caller on to local services, within Jewish Care or in the wider community, or if further support is required, refer them to a member of Jewish Care's Community Support and Social Work team (a free service), who will then arrange to talk to them or meet them to discuss their specific needs further. If support is needed for the carer, a separate referral can be made to the Family Carers Team. People are supported and guided on how to access support from the NHS and local authorities. They will also be supported to find out more about Jewish Care's dementia services and other organisations and charities.

The Community Support and Social Work (CSSW) team has a specialist dementia team. This team has strong links with local and national services and can provide support in the community to those who are living with dementia. The team also works closely with all Jewish Care's services, especially those for people living with dementia, for example Memory Way Cafes. Following on from the initial contact with the help desk, a member of the CSSW team can call the person back. They may also arrange a visit to have a more in-depth conversation. The CSSW worker can remain in contact with the person for several weeks, months or longer. Often a CSSW worker will have worked with a person from early diagnosis to later stages when the person may seek further care (such as home care or residential care). The service can provide very practical advice on areas such as how to apply for lasting power of attorney and the emotional aspects of living with dementia. Typically, the CSSW worker will support the person to find groups such as Singing for Memory or Memory Way Cafes, day centres, home care, live-in care and residential care. They will often attend reviews with the person and their family carer at the service, for example a review in a care home. A very important part of the CSSW referral process is gathering holistic information about the person and their life. This includes their likes, dislikes, preferences, and a history of their life (if the person is happy to share this information). This life story can be very helpful for professional carers, such as a care-home worker, so that they can relate to the person, bond with them and offer them the kind of care and activities they prefer. It is through good systems for sharing relevant information that the best care and support can be provided.

The Family Carers Team (a free service) is trained to work with carers of people living with dementia. The team is there to support and enable the family member to continue this vital role (if that is their wish). It offers emotional support, practical advice and guidance, information and access to various services, and advocates on the person's behalf to help ensure they receive any assistance to which they are entitled. Often carers will have ongoing support from the support worker over a number of years. It can involve regular telephone support, one-to-one meetings and carers' support groups. The support groups for family carers offer opportunities to talk and share experiences with others supporting their relatives or partners with dementia. Family careers often describe this service as the lifeline that helps them maintain their caring roles. Sometimes they dip in and out of the services but they know they need not be alone and can get access to empathetic and knowledgeable support when needed.

There is a network of other services offered by Jewish Care specifically for people living with dementia, including the following:

- *Memory Way Cafes* offer warm and welcoming environments for informal social gatherings for people living with dementia, together with their family carers. Some cafes meet monthly and some every second week. Formats vary, but they usually meet in a communal building. They are normally run by trained volunteers who are supported by a community dementia worker. Good company, refreshments and topical discussions are on offer and one-to-one advice can also be given. Sometimes people prefer to come to the cafes instead of more formal or structured services such as day centres. Often members of the cafes form relationships with other people living with dementia or family members and they exchange contact details and keep in contact between cafes. People describe this as a very important aspect of the cafes that helps greatly to reduce a sense of isolation.
- *Singing for Memory groups* offer singing sessions that also provide a stimulating social environment, bringing together people who are living with dementia, and their carers. They have similar formats to the Memory Way Cafes. The unique feature of these groups is the singing sessions where the members develop a repertoire of

songs and combine it with movement and gentle exercise. They aim to increase wellbeing, as well as giving opportunities for social engagement and mutual support. People often sing songs relating to Jewish festivals and traditional music and songs. This can generate shared memories from childhood and early life and often reinforces a sense of belonging and a shared cultural identity. Singing for Memory groups and Memory Way Cafes have a strong relationship-centred focus. They help build on a sense of security and continuity with members. Over time, people develop bonds with the group and a sense of belonging. People often report a sense of purpose and fulfilment because they have been able to support other members and share experiences with them. The groups often give people opportunities to share past experiences relating to work, family, childhood, music and song. This strengthens a sense of identity, significance and a feeling that one matters as a person.

- Jewish Care runs three *day centres for people living with dementia* that are open Monday to Friday. They have an average attendance of 22 people living with dementia per day. The centres offer people support in decision making, and using their capacity for choice, along with developing strategies to live with their dementia. All of the centres celebrate Jewish festivals, for example, a Seder service at Passover or Rosh Hashanah events for the Jewish New Year. They also celebrate Jewish traditions such as Shabbat kiddush (prayers) and candle lighting on Fridays. This allows people to maintain their Jewish cultural heritage and to feel part of a warm community. People often attend day centres for several years from relatively early stage dementia to later stages. Jewish Care decided to continue to run these dementia day centres at a time when local authorities and other organisations have phased them out. Jewish Care takes the view that these services are highly valued by people living with dementia, and their family carers. They are often described by family members as the services that have enabled the person living with dementia to remain at home. Local authority funding for day centre placements has diminished greatly in the past six years. Previously, in some boroughs, funding was not means tested and the threshold of need was lower. In Jewish Care, the majority of members are self-funding but the organisation subsidises each place by over 50 per cent. The continuance of this service is judged to reflect the organisation's commitment to supporting people living with dementia to live well in the community.

- Jewish Care's *Home Care service* is designed to offer members of the Jewish community the support they require to live independently in their own home from staff who are trained to understand their culture and traditions. Maintaining kosher laws about food is very important for many of Jewish Care's service users. Therefore, in their kitchens and dining rooms they will frequently have separate utensils and crockery for milk and meat dishes (they do not mix them). They may also strictly observe rules about resting on Saturdays and other major festivals. For a person living with dementia, these traditions and faith-based practices can often be central to their sense of identity and an understanding of this, on the part of the carer, can be vital – it can avoid unnecessary stress and help maintain a sense of belonging and wellbeing. Over time, home care workers can develop a person-centred knowledge about what is important to the person, including their faith and traditions. Culturally familiar words and phrases can also make a difference and help a person feel safe, for example wishing a person 'mazel tov' (congratulations) on the bar mitzvah of their grandson. Jewish Care has a culture of sharing and inviting staff to join in Jewish traditions and holds this as vital to providing services that are specific and bespoke for the Jewish community. The majority of home care hours are spent on supporting people living with dementia with personal care and light housework. However, some clients also request one-to-one support with activities to keep stimulated, such as cognitive stimulation therapy, and the organisation has trained some home care workers to do this.

- Jewish Care runs nine *residential and nursing homes* that provide services for people living with dementia. Its care and nursing homes have been refurbished, redeveloped or purpose built using up-to-date dementia design principles to enhance the quality of life for people living with dementia. Care and nursing staff receive ongoing dementia training. The care staff receive dementia qualifications through the Qualifications and Credit Framework and this is enhanced through in-house dementia training and mentoring provided by the Arts, Disability and Dementia Team (see Strategic Aim 3 below for a full description of this team's strategy). The staff are also trained in end-of-life care and we work to ensure people can live well with dementia up to the end of life and so die in a familiar Jewish environment.

Jewish Care's residential and nursing homes offer a Jewish environment as described above. They tend to be community hubs for the families and friends of the residents. Four of the homes have been built on a campus model where there is space for community gatherings, cafe/dining facilities and community centres and dementia day centres. Strong links are developed with local schools and synagogues. Rabbis and congregants are encouraged to visit the homes and make sure people living in the homes maintain contact with their faith community. Work placements from the schools are very welcome and mother and baby visits are a very popular feature on the home's activities programme. Volunteers are a very important feature of life in the home. It is a very strong tradition in the Jewish community to volunteer and give time and skills to charitable causes. Volunteers can be found in Jewish Care homes, running groups and activities, outings, befriending and supporting at meal times. They are a vital link with the community and often join local fundraising committees to support the homes.

Jewish Care is committed to improving and developing relationship-centred care and seeking out new approaches. The occupational therapist has been implementing an approach to dementia that is widely used in the United States, Australia and Europe but is still relatively unknown in the UK. This is the Montessori Inspired Lifestyle, which was developed by Cameron J. Camp (n.d.) based on the pioneering work of Maria Montessori in the early 20th century in education methods for children. It focuses on the individual's strengths and sensory-stimulating environments. In dementia care homes, the Montessori Inspired Lifestyle aims to create resident-driven communities where the abilities, interests and preferences of people living with dementia are respected, maximised and encouraged.

- Jewish Care's *independent living apartments* offer rental housing with care from an on-site support team and aim to support people to live independently if/when they develop dementia. At the point of taking an apartment, most residents do not have a diagnosis of dementia. However, a significant proportion of residents will go on to develop dementia. Jewish Care's independent living teams and the wider care and support teams within the organisation aim to support the person living with dementia to live independently, in their apartment, for as long as possible and if they need/want to move into a higher level of residential or nursing care, that can be provided on the same campus or locally. Currently, Jewish Care has one independent living scheme (45 residents) based in a community campus in Golders Green (London) alongside a dementia care home and a community centre. It is located in a vibrant Jewish area with many kosher shops and restaurants. The majority of the residents living there are Holocaust survivors or refugees. Jewish Care is currently developing two more independent living schemes in the London area (to accommodate 32 and 45 residents). Demand for this kind of accommodation is growing. As with the other services described above, residents articulate the benefits of living in a culturally and faith-specific service with a sense of community and belonging. They also appreciate locations that are geographically located in areas with strong Jewish communities and facilities.

Strategic aim 3: Ensuring our service users consistently high quality from the onset of dementia to the end of life

Jewish Care is committed to enhancing the way it serves Jewish people with dementia and their families, ensuring they receive quality support that reflects emerging good practice and new ways of working. It strives to develop its workforce to achieve core skills and knowledge in dementia care, creating a pathway that ensures people with dementia and their carers receive culturally sensitive services that enable and involve them as partners in care at all stages of the condition.

Since 2012, Jewish Care has had a dedicated team to support staff development across the organisation in dementia care. The team is the Arts, Disability and Dementia Team (ADDT). Their learning and development strategy aims to develop core competencies as follows:

- *Relationship-centred approach* – to work to equip staff and volunteers to engage with the people using Jewish Care's services and to build relationships with them on an equal basis as people. This involves good communication, empathy, active listening, being able to put yourself in the place of the other person, and building community (working collaboratively with the person and supporting that person to engage with their communities). It encompasses an awareness of how to support and encourage the relationships between people (according to the individual's wishes), creating opportunities for people to live and participate in communities and to be enabled and empowered to contribute to them. This is the opposite of a task-focused approach and involves a cultural shift from that way of working.

- *Resourcefulness and creativity* – working with staff and volunteers to be in tune within their own resourcefulness and have confidence within it. In practice, this involves being confident to recognise and focus on the needs of the people using Jewish Care's services, including mental health and wellbeing. It means being able to use that creativity relating to the people who use the services, including building spontaneous opportunities for fun and bringing forth a meaningful life. Jewish Care values the personality and caring nature of its staff and volunteers and the way that these characteristics can enhance the experience of the people who use our services.

  Creativity is not only about taking part in arts activities, it is also about breaking away from the way things are usually done by using new approaches. A participatory arts approach can be applied to a one-to-one session or a group and is facilitated rather than directed by the creative practitioner. The facilitator takes the direction from the person with dementia, starting where they are. The activity focuses on the person's strengths, not on dementia or disability. Choice for each participant is provided at a level suited to that individual. Everyone's contribution is valued. Participation in the activity can be verbal or non-verbal, sensory or just observation. It is during the process of an activity where meaningful connections are made and memory and creativity can be nourished and expressed.

- *Delivering an enabling culture of care* – working with staff and volunteers so that their approaches support and strengthen the abilities of service users and reduce their limitations. They recognise that the person is at the heart and they are driving their support services. It is about empowering the person to achieve what they want and inspiring them to reach their full potential. Staff and volunteers must seek to identify and understand what the person can do and work creatively to enhance this. In this context, it is essential to be able to recognise and to have good strategies to respond to impairments such as sight loss, hearing loss and agnosia (inability to interpret sensations and hence to recognize things, typically as a result of brain damage) so that the person can still adapt and achieve what they would like to do.

- *Responding to psychological, emotional, cultural and spiritual needs* – staff are developed and supported to recognise that loneliness and isolation are often associated with dementia and disabilities. They are equipped to address and respond to emotional and psychological needs and to see that these are as important as support with physical needs. Sometimes this also involves reconciling individual needs with communal living and an understanding and ability to respond to the interpersonal and social nature of our environments.

- *Skills for reflective practice* – being with staff and volunteers on their journey of learning and professional development through reflective practice is crucial. Relationship-focused and person-centred care is a continuous learning journey as this approach is individual to each person. Staff and volunteers are supported through reflective practice – establishing and building on good working practices to improve quality of life (this includes processes, standards and documentation).

Supporting people living with dementia and their spiritual lives

Jewish Care values the rights of people living with dementia to live their faith and cultural traditions. Supporting people to live well with dementia often brings unexpected and surprising rewards. Rabbi Cary Kozberg (n.d.) writes:

Dementia may steal the mind but it cannot encroach upon the soul. In my work I see how alive and vibrant the soul can remain, even when a person's cognitive capacities are significantly diminished. This is because God addresses each person in the way he or she is able to hear, as Midrash Tanhuma affirms: 'The voice of the Eternal is in the strength – that is, fitted to the strength, the ability – of each and every person: men according to their abilities, women according to their abilities, and young according to their abilities, the elderly according to their abilities.' As I've learned…sometimes the soul can hear the

Voice even better, and respond more spontaneously when the mind no longer gets in the way.

Jewish Care's services are open to anybody who identifies as Jewish, regardless of their affiliation to a synagogue or branch of Judaism. It works with and welcomes support from the synagogues' welfare and spiritual leaders. The organisation employs a chaplain but in addition to him many community rabbis visit the homes and centres and provide pastoral support to people living with dementia, and their family carers. In care homes, residents living with dementia are supported to take part in family-style Friday night Shabbat prayers and suppers. On Saturdays, the homes have community rabbis and/or volunteers leading Shabbat services. All of the Jewish festivals are celebrated in the homes and centres run by Jewish Care and provide a timeline and sense of purpose, identity and continuity that is often extremely beneficial for people living with dementia. The sense of belonging to a community, faith and tradition can remain strong for people living with dementia and can be reinforced by familiar prayers, hymns and rituals.

People now tend to come in to live in care and nursing homes much closer to end of life than in previous years. They tend to live in their own homes or in supported accommodation for longer. Care and nursing staff in Jewish Care's homes work to ensure that people with dementia have the right spiritual support at the end of life. The person's wishes are recorded in advance and they work closely with the person's rabbi to ensure their death is cared for according to their particular Judaic customs and practice.

Spirituality is a personal choice and people see and live it in unique and individual ways. Jewish Care follows a person-centred approach to spirituality. They are guided by the service user and seek to respond to their needs and requests. The organisation is careful to respect people's diversity and strives to be sensitive to the rights of all people living with dementia.

Linda and Ron's story: A Jewish couple living with dementia

Ron (aged 85) was diagnosed with mild to moderate Alzheimer's disease four years ago, though the signs were apparent two years prior to this. Since that time, his wife and main carer (Linda), says that 'everything has changed'.

Linda is from Birmingham and the couple met in London when she was 24. They were introduced at a function by a friend from Birmingham and married in June 1965 in Linda's synagogue. Linda worked as a part-time secretary and Ron was a chartered accountant.

Linda stopped working when they had their first daughter and Ron continued working until his late seventies. They have two daughters and three grandchildren.

Ron has had cancer and has a number of other long-term conditions. He continues to live with Alzheimer's disease, with very poor short-term memory and confusion.

After the diagnosis four years ago, Ron's two daughters applied for power of attorney over both Linda's and Ron's health and finances. He also was written to by the Driver and Vehicle Licensing Agency (DVLA) and stopped driving.

Linda and Ron are both members of a synagogue and used to attend together every Shabbat. Since Ron's Alzheimer's diagnosis, he has given up going to synagogue as it became too difficult for him. He used to go to the synagogue every day for Shabbat morning service to make a minyan (ten men) and lay tefillin (a set of small black leather boxes containing scrolls of parchment inscribed with verses from the Torah prayer) but shortly after his diagnosis he also stopped doing this. Linda still finds this difficult to accept as he was the one insistent on going to the synagogue. However, he still says Kiddush (prayers) every Friday evening with Linda and sometimes at his daughter's home. Ron also reads perfectly from the Haggadah (order of service) at the family Pesach (Passover meal).

On his 80th birthday, Ron did read Maftir (Maftir is the concluding section of the portion of the Torah chanted or read in a Jewish service on the Sabbath and festivals *and* the person who recites the blessings before and after the chanting or reading of this section) in synagogue and had his second bar mitzvah at the age of 83.

Ron was the treasurer for many years of the local Israel group but again had to give this up following his diagnosis as the role became too much for him.

For the last 18 months, Ron has attended a Jewish day centre twice a week. Linda feels that this is good stimulation for Ron, who otherwise sits at home and watches television. It also gives her a much-needed break from her caring role. They also both attend a Jewish Memory Way Cafe as often as possible. Linda was also referred for family carer's support at Jewish Care and she has had an allocated worker since September 2017. They meet monthly for practical help and advice and emotional support in her caring role.

Linda still enjoys going to the synagogue on Saturdays, but now is unable to leave Ron alone. She was referred to the local carers' centre where she had a carer's assessment. The outcome has been an award of £24 per week to be given as a direct payment for her to buy in some care on a Saturday morning to enable her to continue to go the synagogue. She plans to use Jewish Care's home care to provide this service. She has also been encouraged to refer Ron for a needs-led assessment via social services with a view to him having a care package to help her with some of Ron's care.

Linda was a committee member at her synagogue (Chesed – a 'chesed institution' in modern Judaism may refer to any charitable organization run by religious Jewish groups or individuals. i.e. it's a description of the 'religious devotion' of the committee so Jewish Care is 'chesed' by definition and its committee members are held to be compassionate ('chesed')) and has had to give up her involvement with this since Ron's diagnosis of dementia. She explained that many members of the synagogue and committee used to visit regularly, but a number of them have stopped over the past few years. There are a couple who still contact her and this contact is very important. The rabbi's visits to Ron are very important to help him lay tefillin, and Linda has asked him to keep coming even if Ron's condition deteriorates, as it is a very important part of his identity. They still receive the weekly synagogue newsletter and are invited to events by the Chesed committee. Linda plans to attend the Chanukah tea with Ron next month. Keeping contact with the synagogue and feeling part of the community remains very important to them and helps them feel emotionally stronger.

Linda is supported by her two daughters and would like to continue looking after Ron. She will be 80 next year.

References

Camp, C. (n.d.) Centre for Applied Research in Dementia. Available at: www.cen4ard.com/index.php?option=com_content&view=article&id=63&Itemid=191 [accessed 15/03/2018].

Department of Health (2009) *Living Well with Dementia: A National Strategy.* Available from: www.gov.uk/government/uploads/system/uploads/attachment_data/file/168220/dh_094051.pdf [accessed 05/01/2018].

Kitwood, T. (1997) *Dementia Reconsidered: The Person Comes First.* Buckingham: Open University Press.

Kozberg, Rabbi C. (n.d.) *A Jewish Response to Dementia: Honoring Broken Tablets.* Available at: www.caregiverslibrary.org/portals/0/Microsoft%20Word%20-%20A%20Jewish%20Response%20to%20Dementia[1].pdf [accessed 05/012018].

Nolan, M.R., Brown, J., Davies, S., Nolan, J. and Keady, J. (2006) *The Senses Framework: Improving care for older people through a relationship-centred approach.* Getting Research into Practice (GRiP) Report No 2. Available at: https://shura.shu.ac.uk/280/1/PDF_Senses [accessed 15/03/2018].

CHAPTER 7

Dementia, Rights and Black, Asian and Minority Ethnic Communities

Toby Williamson

Introduction

Considering dementia through the lens of rights, especially human rights, is a perspective that has generated increasing interest in recent years. This view includes the development of policy and practice in dementia care using rights-based approaches which incorporate the voices of people with dementia, and their carers. Yet much less attention has been paid to the rights of particular groups in the population affected by dementia, including people from Black, Asian and minority ethnic (BAME) communities. This chapter considers the relevance of rights-based approaches, especially human rights, to dementia care and the lives of people affected by dementia from BAME communities.

The chapter starts off by describing different legal frameworks that provide rights to people with dementia, then reviews recent literature that considers rights in relation to people with dementia, especially those from BAME communities. It goes on to look at rights-based approaches in policy and practice and how these relate to people with dementia from BAME communities. Before concluding, the chapter considers three scenarios exploring rights in relation to people with dementia from BAME communities. The chapter ends with some key messages about dementia, rights and BAME communities.

Rights and dementia

'Rights' is a term that many people use in relation to what they believe services should be providing to them, their relatives or their friends. Practitioners may also use or encounter the term, sometimes with trepidation for fear of applying the law incorrectly, and it is also frequently used in discussions and debates by policy makers, influencers and opinion formers. Rights come in many forms and 'rights' as a term can be used in generic and non-specific ways. Rights can refer to several different legal frameworks and conventions and it is not always clear what is being referred to when the term is used. It is therefore helpful to briefly define what the term includes, both in respect of dementia and the experiences of people from BAME communities.

Rights may be used to describe:

- rights to public services
- rights to make decisions
- rights for people subject to compulsory detention and/or treatment
- rights protecting people from discrimination
- human rights.

Rights to public services

Having citizenship of a country usually entitles someone to have the right to access a range of public services. These are covered by numerous laws and statutes and can include the right to health, education, social care, housing, welfare benefits and pensions. Yet while some of these rights may be unconditional, others are not, and this can be the source of confusion and frustration for many people, including those affected by dementia.

An example of this is in the UK where there is a universal right to free healthcare at the point of need but rights to publicly funded social care, housing, and welfare benefits are conditional depending on the financial situation of the individual and the severity of need (the conditions also vary between the four nations that make up the UK). So a person may be diagnosed with dementia and receive free healthcare for the medical aspects of the condition but not be entitled to any publicly funded social care for the social needs that arise from the condition, including the need for residential care. The requirement to pay for care out of one's own bank account or having to sell assets, including the house one owns, can frequently come as a shock to people.

Understanding one's rights to public services can therefore be a complicated task, even where a single law covers access to services. For example, legislative reform in the UK of laws and statutes covering the rights to publicly funded social care resulted in the introduction of the Care Act 2014, covering England, although devolution means that different (though similar) pieces of legislation cover Wales, Scotland and Northern Ireland. To give some idea of the Act's complexity, it runs to 251 pages and the statutory guidance to the Act issued in 2014 is over 400 pages and was further revised in 2017 (Department of Health 2014).

As other chapters in this book have indicated, people from BAME communities and their families experience a number of difficulties accessing health and social care services. Some of the reasons for these difficulties are common to people with dementia from all communities but some are specific to people from BAME communities. People living with dementia from BAME communities and their carers are entitled to care, support and treatment that is available, accessible, culturally sensitive, responsive and appropriate. Services, practitioners and other staff need to ensure that this is provided in the local areas they serve. Irrespective of race or ethnicity, people have the same rights to services as the rest of the population. The barriers and difficulties in accessing public services encountered by BAME people with dementia described in this book may constitute a breach of their rights, and the rights of their families and communities.

However, it should be noted that in many countries, including the UK, rights to services may be more complicated where the immigration status of people means they are not eligible for public funds or publicly funded services. This can apply to asylum seekers and people whose legal right to stay in the country is not clear, perhaps because they have inadvertently stayed beyond what their visa permits (e.g. a relative with dementia visiting family in the UK who deteriorates and needs to stay to receive care) or immigration rules have changed (*The Guardian* 2018).

Where barriers or difficulties encountered by people with dementia from BAME communities and their carers discriminate on the basis of race or ethnicity, it can become a broader issue that draws on wider, rights-based legislation, most notably the Equality Act 2010 in the UK (see below).

Rights to make decisions

People with conditions such as dementia that cause cognitive impairments also have rights regarding their ability to make decisions. The Mental Capacity Act (MCA) 2005 in England and Wales (and similar legislation in Scotland and Northern Ireland) involves a framework of principles, processes and safeguards to support people who have conditions affecting their ability to make decisions. It empowers people to make decisions for themselves wherever possible, enables people to plan ahead for a time when they may not be able to make decisions, and has a 'best interests' process to enable decisions to be made on their behalf if they are unable to do so themselves.

However, there is considerable evidence to indicate that some health and social care practitioners have insufficient awareness and understanding of the MCA (Williams *et al.* 2014; House of Lords 2014). This can result in people's rights to make decisions for themselves, or protecting them when decisions are made on their behalf, not being upheld.

Furthermore, family carers do not have unconditional rights under the MCA to make decisions on behalf of a person who lacks capacity to make a decision. This may come as an unwelcome surprise for some families where a relative has dementia. Tensions can arise where dementia practitioners are supporting a person with dementia to make a decision or making a decision on their behalf that their family disagrees with, around issues such as safeguarding or a move into residential care. Furthermore, people with more severe dementia may make decisions or act in ways that break with their religious beliefs or customs, such as no longer adhering to prohibitions on certain food. Discerning the effect of their dementia on a person's right and ability to self-determine against adherence to rules or customs may prove very complicated. A report on the initial impact of the MCA on BAME communities found significant issues concerning awareness, understanding and accessibility of the MCA, decision-making processes in families not reflecting the process described in the MCA (or the assumptions of some health and social care practitioners), and difficulties engaging with the MCA reflecting wider difficulties for BAME people engaging with health and social care services (Mental Health Foundation 2008).

Rights for people subject to compulsory detention and/or treatment

Many jurisdictions have laws allowing people with a mental disorder (including dementia) to be admitted, detained, treated and cared for in hospital or registered nursing homes for their own safety or the safety of others when they lack the capacity to consent to this. This legislation includes legal protections for the person who is subject to the requirements of the legislation.

Both the Mental Health Act (MHA) 1983 and the MCA in England and Wales (and similar legislation in Scotland and Northern Ireland) authorise compulsory detention and treatment. Under Article 5 of the Human Rights Act, people are entitled to a number of legal safeguards because detention under these laws constitute a deprivation of liberty prohibited by the Article unless those safeguards are in place. These safeguards include a legal process that authorises the process of admission, detention, care and tretament, a right of appeal and a right to advocacy.

The MHA tends not to be used for people with dementia but the Deprivation of Liberty Safeguards (DoLS) that are part of the MCA are frequently used for people with dementia in care homes. In 2015–16, 76,530 applications for DoLS were authorised in England, the vast majority of which were for people with dementia in care homes (NHS Digital 2016). DoLS have generated considerable controversy, partly because of their bureaucratic complexity, and there are proposals to simplify them. It is interesting to note that while detentions under the MHA of African-Caribbean people, especially young men, attracts a lot of critical attention, the same concern are not expressed about the much greater number of older people detained in care homes and subject to DoLS.

While the MHA and DoLS apply human rights and safeguards for people with dementia, their powers of detention and compulsory care, as well as their complexity, may generate concern and even fear among people from BAME communities, especially those who have family or friends with experience of compulsory detention and treatment under the MHA.

Rights protecting people from discrimination

Particular groups in society who have experienced unfair treatment or discrimination based on ignorance, prejudice or hostility have rights and legal protection in the UK under the Equality Act 2010. The Equality Act defines the groups afforded rights under the Act in terms of 'protected characteristics'. These are: age, disability, gender reassignment, race (including 'colour, nationality, ethnic or national origin'), religion or belief, sex, sexual orientation, marriage and civil partnership, and pregnancy and maternity. It protects people from discrimination based on any of these characteristics in the workplace and in wider society, such as the provision of goods and services, including health, social care and housing.

The Equality Act is clearly important in protecting people from BAME communities from racism and other forms of discrimination. And for BAME people with dementia it provides other legal protections. Because dementia is a condition most people experience in later life, the Act can provide protection against ageism but also ensure that people with young onset dementia are not excluded from services. Furthermore, where the impairments caused by dementia have a 'substantial' and 'long-term negative effect' on a person's ability to do 'normal daily activities', they would constitute a disability under the Act (HM Government 2010, p.4). Some people may not want to define their dementia as a disability but this doesn't exclude them from the protections provided by the Act.

How far legislation like the Equality Act has benefited disabled people and people from BAME communities is difficult to measure. It can certainly be argued that society has become more tolerant and inclusive of many groups protected by this legislation and there is less overt racism expressed towards many BAME groups, for example. Yet employment rates for disabled people have remained consistently well below employment rates for people without disabilities and the current hostility and suspicion expressed towards many Muslims and migrants indicates that prejudice and bigotry are still very much alive. The Equality and Human Rights Commission in England published a large range of research reports looking at the impact of legislation and the experiences of groups covered by the Equality Act.[1]

The Act also uses what is known as a 'social model of disability'. The model began to emerge in the 1970s although the term was not coined until the 1980s (Oliver and Sapey 2012). Broadly speaking, the model defines disability not in relation to the individual but in terms of how society responds to people with impairments (which can be physical, sensory, mental or cognitive) caused by health conditions. Whereas a biomedical model of disability locates the problem in the individual and focuses on providing them with treatment and interventions to cure or 'fix' the problem, the social model defines disability in terms of the attitudes, behaviours, processes and environments of wider society which create the obstacles and barriers to the participation of people with impairments. A focus on rights, changing attitudes, physical environments and making 'reasonable adjustments' to working practices becomes the focus of activity under the social model.

Variations to the model have been proposed more recently to take more into account the individual's experience of living with impairments and the impact these have on the person. These have generated discussion and debate. In some respects, the move to develop 'dementia-friendly communities' (DFCs) in many countries around the world is an example of the social model in action, although DFCs tend not to challenge the biomedical view of dementia or be framed in reference to disability rights (Williamson 2016).

---

1   www.equalityhumanrights.com/en

Human rights

Human rights formally arrived in the UK with the Human Rights Act 1998 which, in effect, put the European Convention on Human Rights (ECHR) onto the UK statute books. The ECHR contains a number of rights (known as 'Articles') relevant to people with dementia and people from BAME communities. These include:

- *Article 2* – the right to life (with virtually no exceptions).
- *Article 3* – prohibits inhuman or degrading treatment or punishment (with no exceptions or limitations).
- *Article 5* – everyone has the right to liberty and security of person (subject to lawful arrest or detention, which can include people with mental disorders).
- *Article 8* – the right to private and family life (subject to certain restrictions that are 'in accordance with the law' and 'necessary in a democratic society').
- *Article 14* – freedom from discrimination, including on the grounds of race, colour [sic], national or social origin, or association with national minority disability 'or other status'.

Respecting the lives of people with dementia, even when they are in the very last stages of the illness and receiving palliative care, showing dignity and respect when providing care and treatment, not placing unnecessary restrictions on a person just because they have dementia, and respecting their privacy and their family relationships, are all actions others need to take to uphold the human rights of people with dementia. Article 14 is particularly important for BAME people affected by dementia as it prohibits discrimination in the implementation of any of the other articles.

However, the Human Rights Act and the ECHR make no mention of disability[2] or rights to public services. The United Nations Universal Declaration of Human Rights only mentions disability once and in order therefore to make human rights relevant to people with disabilities, the United Nations adopted the Convention on the Rights of Persons with Disabilities in 2006 (UNCRPD). It has been ratified by 175 countries including the UK

---

2   The European Court of Human Rights has ruled that Article 14's reference to 'other status' includes disability. The ECHR does use the rather archaic and pejorative term 'unsound mind' to describe people with mental disorder, including dementia, who can lawfully be deprived of their liberty under Article 5.

(which means governments should ensure their country's compliance with the Convention).

The UNCRPD is based on a 'human rights model of disability'. This is a development of the social model of disability that partly builds on the social model but makes explicit reference to human rights and equalities.[3] It defines people with impairments as equal citizens ('rights holders') and others (e.g. health and social care practitioners) as having duties and responsibilities towards them as citizens ('duty holders'). The UNCRPD has 50 articles and key articles relevant to people with dementia are listed in Table 7.1 at the end of this chapter. A number of the articles emphasise access to services, citizenship rights and the opportunity to participate in society on an equal basis with people without disabilities. The preamble to the Convention also states that countries ratifying the Convention are:

> concerned about the difficult conditions faced by persons with disabilities who are subject to multiple or aggravated forms of discrimination on the basis of race, colour, sex, language, religion, political or other opinion, national, ethnic, indigenous or social origin, property, birth, age or other status. (United Nations 2006, p.2)

With its emphasis on access and positive rights to services, combined with the recognition of additional or multiple discrimination, the UNCRPD represents an important legal framework to both protect and promote the rights of BAME people affected by dementia.

Despite the importance of human rights and the UNCRPD, people can find it difficult to understand how they might apply in practice other than through complicated legal processes. To try and overcome this difficulty, practical frameworks have been developed to support human rights-based approaches in the development and provision of services, and the relevance of those rights to people who use services. Two such examples are given in the box below.

---

3   A useful summary of different models of disability can be found on Alzheimer Europe's website (Gove, *et al.* 2017)

PANEL
(Participation, Accountability, Non-Discrimination and Equality, Empowerment, Legality) principles (adapted from the Scottish Human Rights Commission 2009)

Participation	People with disabilities can participate in decisions affecting their human rights
Accountability	There is monitoring of organisations' adherence to human rights affecting people with disabilities and remedial action taken where necessary
Non-discrimination and equality	All forms of discrimination and unfair treatment of people with disabilities are prohibited
Empowerment	People with disabilities are given the information and support necessary to enable them to participate in decision making and claiming their rights
Legality	Rights are recognised as legally enforceable entitlements by public authorities

FREDA	The following principles should be
(Fairness, Respect, Equality, Dignity, Autonomy) principles	embedded in everyday professional practice in relation to patients:
A human rights-based approach to healthcare (Curtice and Exworthy 2010)	Fairness
	Respect
	Equality
	Dignity
	Autonomy

Examples of putting these principles into practice include:

- the formation of a network of influencing and campaigning groups actively involving or led by people with dementia as part of the Dementia Engagement and Empowerment Project (DEEP)[4]

---

4   http://dementiavoices.org.uk

- a successful campaign involving people with dementia to get the UK government to review the eligibility criteria for disabled car parking permits to include people with cognitive impairments
- the formation of the Dementia Alliance on Culture and Ethnicity to raise awareness of dementia in BAME communities and the services that support them[5]
- the development of community dementia action alliances, many of which include BAME community organisations
- a range of involvement guides developed by people with dementia including ones on language and terminology, employment, research, accessible information and events.[6]

Equalities, rights, dementia and ethnicity

In terms of written evidence there has been a growing focus on rights and equalities and people with dementia from BAME communities. As can be seen elsewhere in this book, there is a substantial body of literature exploring many aspects of dementia as it affects people from different BAME communities. Yet explicit considerations of the links between dementia, ethnicity and rights have been somewhat sporadic.

In 2010, the Joseph Rowntree Foundation published a review of equality and diversity issues for older people with high support needs including dementia, which raised the issue of human rights in connection with dementia and referred to problems experienced by BAME people with dementia in terms of their rights to services (Blood and Bamford 2010). The following year, Age UK published a guide for practitioners and commissioners of services for older people on equality and human rights, although this made little mention of dementia (Age UK 2011). An evidence review published by Age UK on diversity in older people and access to services considered both people with dementia and older BAME people but it identified no publications which looked at the two together within the parameters of the report (Moriarty and Manthorpe 2012). The House of Commons All-Party Parliamentary Group on Dementia in England published a report on the experience of people with dementia from BAME communities but this focused on access to services and made no mention of rights (All-Party Parliamentary Group on

---

5   www.demace.com

6   http://dementiavoices.org.uk/resources/deep-guides

Dementia 2013). A more explicit focus linking rights, dementia and BAME communities featured in the 2016 publication, *Dementia, Equity and Rights*, which included a number of recommendations for service commissioners and providers to ensure BAME people affected by dementia could exercise their rights to services (Voluntary Organisations Disability Group 2016). Truswell, writing in 2018, commented on the difficulty of embedding human rights in healthcare for migrant and BAME communities affected by dementia and ways these difficulties could be addressed (Truswell 2018).

Rights-based approaches in dementia

Although public discourses about dementia rarely link it with disability and human rights, McGettrick points out that discussion of those links goes back to the 1990s (McGettrick 2015). Yet, taking England as an example, dementia policy has generally been slow on the uptake of a rights-based approach. One could argue that a succession of national strategies on dementia are implicit in emphasising the rights of people with dementia and carers to services they need. These policies have contained some references to these rights as well as human rights but they tend to be buried in the text of the documents and human rights are not the principles which shape the documents.[7] Although the documents do mention BAME people with dementia in terms of rights to services, references to equalities are limited.

An important boost to the human rights and dementia discourse was heralded by the publication of *Dementia, Rights and the Social Model of Disability* (McGettrick 2015). This made the links between equalities and other legal frameworks, the UNCRPD and dementia. It emphasised the importance of involving people with dementia in a human-rights-based approach and this was supported by the work of groups of people with dementia that were part of the DEEP network. In 2016, DEEP published a guide to rights including human rights for people with dementia (Hare 2016) and evidence was submitted to the UN committee responsible for the UNCRPD (Alzheimer's Society 2017; Dementia Policy Think Tank, DEEP Network, Innovations in Dementia Community Interest Company 2017).

---

7   The first National Dementia Strategy refers to 'protecting their [people with dementia and their carers] human rights' (Department of Health 2009, p.49). The Prime Minster's Challenge on Dementia 2020 refers to 'bolstering the human rights of people with dementia' in the context of working with the United Nations independent expert on the human rights of older people (Department of Health 2015, p.20)

Research has been undertaken regarding human rights and dementia using the FREDA principles (Butchard and Kinderman 2017) and there have been joint publications about disability and dementia involving people with dementia and disability activists and writers (Dementia Alliance International 2016; Shakespeare, Zeilig and Mittler 2017).

However, despite the increased focus on rights, these documents are limited in their references to people affected by dementia from BAME communities, and the involvement of BAME people in developing them has been limited. In this respect, the emergence of groups like the Dementia Alliance on Culture and Ethnicity is important as a way of potentially linking ethnicity and rights in dementia care.

In 2015, the Alzheimer's Society in England expressed its support for a rights-based approach to the treatment of people with dementia. This refers to both human rights and the Equality Act and includes a specific call for improved support for people from BAME communities (Alzheimer Society 2015).

Scotland – a human-rights-based approach to dementia and ethnicity

Scotland has had a much more established and explicit focus on social justice and human rights in the development and delivery of public policy than other parts of the UK. This has included its National Strategy on Dementia, and in 2009 a Charter of Rights for People with Dementia and their Carers in Scotland was published, produced by the Cross-Party Group in the Scottish Parliament on Alzheimer's, with Alzheimer Scotland and members of the Scottish Dementia Working Group, made up of people with dementia (Alzheimer Scotland 2009). This was based on the PANEL principles, which are a fundamental part of the human rights-based approach that Scotland has applied to its policies on dementia.

The Charter only briefly mentions ethnicity; it declares that 'people with dementia and their carers have the right to be free from discrimination based on any ground such as age, disability, gender, race, sexual orientation, religious beliefs, social or other status' (Alzheimer Scotland 2009). However, Scotland's second National Strategy on Dementia acknowledged that translating a human-rights-based approach from policy into practice has proved challenging in Scotland especially in relation to equalities (Scottish Government 2013). The strategy led to a report from Scotland's National Advisory Group on

Dementia and Equality which identified 17 commitments under a human-rights-based approach on which to address issues of equalities and dementia (Watchman 2016).

Three examples of dementia, rights and people from BAME communities

To illustrate how different rights might apply to people with dementia from BAME communities, here are three examples.

Cheryl

Cheryl is a 50-year-old woman of African-Caribbean heritage with Down syndrome. She also has diabetes and quite severe visual impairments. Cheryl lives in specialist supported housing for people with learning disabilities, where she has a key worker. Her mother and sister live nearby and Cheryl goes to visit them every day; they are a very important part of Cheryl's life. They help Cheryl make a lot of decisions. Cheryl also has a social worker from a community learning disability team. The social worker has helped Cheryl's mother to support Cheryl in making more decisions about how she spends her money, rather than making decisions on Cheryl's behalf.

Recently, Cheryl has become very forgetful and confused; she has got lost on three occasions travelling on journeys that previously she had been very familiar with. Her ability to look after herself has also deteriorated significantly. Cheryl's mother and sister are very worried and want her to have more support where she lives. Cheryl's key worker thinks it 'may be just a phase that Cheryl is going through' and has said that Cheryl's mother is 'over-involved' and getting 'over-emotional'. However, the key worker (who is not African-Caribbean) also mentions that if things don't change then the family might have to look after Cheryl or that Cheryl might need to go into residential care for people with learning disabilities. Cheryl's mother and sister don't want either of these options.

The social worker suggests that Cheryl perhaps needs to go to see her GP as this may help.

Commentary and key points

- *Diagnosing dementia* – Although the prevalence of dementia among people with learning disabilities is much higher than it is in the rest of the population, it is often not recognised or its effects are put down to the person's learning disability. It is important that learning disability organisations are aware that dementia is likely to affect older people they support and know how to respond if someone is showing signs of it. Although assessing and diagnosing dementia in people with learning disabilities can be challenging, it is the right of someone like Cheryl to be referred to her GP. The social worker's suggestion of Cheryl seeing her GP is important because this should lead to an assessment of Cheryl's health and a possible diagnosis of dementia. Cheryl has a right to be assessed and if she does have dementia she also has a right to be told this, in a way that she can understand. Both Cheryl and her family may need support to come to terms with this.

- *Making decisions* – The response of Cheryl's key worker suggests that they are not aware of the links between learning disability and dementia, and they are insensitive if not prejudiced in their view of Cheryl and her family. This is an issue that needs addressing, probably through staff training and development. Different families and people from different ethnic minority communities may have different ways of communicating and expressing themselves, and reflect different types of inter-dependence. But as with Cheryl's mother, it doesn't mean that the importance of independence isn't also recognised by BAME families affected by dementia. Cheryl's right to make decisions for herself wherever possible must be respected under the MCA, together with the involvement of her family. Article 12 of the UNCRPD emphasises the importance of supporting Cheryl to make her own decisions.

- *Rights to social care* – Cheryl also has a right to have her care and support needs reassessed under the Care Act 2014, and her mother and sister also have the right to a carer's assessment. These assessments should take into account the family's cultural background and needs. This may enable additional support to be provided to Cheryl to allow her to stay living where she is. The underlying principle of the Care Act is the wellbeing of people with care and support needs. The articles in the UNCRPD that promote independent living, participation in the community and access to services reinforce Cheryl's rights as a person with disabilities.

- *Multiple inequalities* – It is also important to recognise that Cheryl potentially experiences multiple inequalities – as a person with disabilities, as a person from an ethnic minority, and as a woman. Disability, race and gender are all 'protected characteristics' under the UK's Equality Act 2010. The Act bans discrimination, harassment and victimisation against people with protected characteristics in employment, education and the provision of goods and services. The learning disability organisation supporting Cheryl needs to be aware of all the protection that the Equality Act provides and not inadvertently discriminate against her if, for example, she is diagnosed with dementia.

Hari

Hari is a 60-year-old Sikh man who grew up in the Punjab in India but came to the UK when he was 14. He works as a delivery driver. His wife died three years ago but he has three sons who all have families. Just before he turned 60 he was diagnosed with early onset Alzheimer's disease having noticed that he was getting confused about everyday things. He told his family about his diagnosis but he does not want his wider circle of friends and colleagues to know. However, his son advises him that he should tell his manager at work. When he does this, the manager immediately responds by saying that he can no longer do his job and will have to resign. Hari also helps out at the temple he attends and when he tells the custodian at the temple about his diagnosis, he is told that he should no longer attend the temple because he might pass on the disease to others. The custodian also tells other people at the temple about Hari's diagnosis.

Three years later, Hari is no longer able to care for himself independently and only speaks in Punjabi, in which none of his sons are fluent. He agrees to go into a local care home but there is only one member of staff who speaks Punjabi and Hari is quite hostile towards three members of staff who are Muslim. The owner of the care home says that he may have to leave.

Commentary and key points
Hari is unusual because he developed Alzheimer's disease at a relatively early age. Because he is in employment and not yet eligible for a state pension,

employment rights and rights to disability benefits are of crucial importance to Hari.

- *Employment rights and rights to welfare benefits* – Under employment rights and equalities legislation it would be illegal to make Hari resign or sack him just because he has been diagnosed with dementia. Hari may have to give up work but if this is on health grounds he should have a proper occupational health assessment (and probably an assessment of his ability to drive) and evidence gathered to show that there is no other job he could do in his workplace given the impairments caused by his dementia. The law requires 'reasonable adjustments' to be made to a person's role to accommodate the impairments caused by a health condition, which can include dementia. If he is getting lost doing deliveries but can still drive the van safely, a reasonable adjustment might be for someone to go with him but this is not reasonable if there are no staff available to do this. An alternative might be to offer him work at the depot if the occupational assessment indicated he could do this. If Hari does have to leave work, he has a right to receive welfare benefits.

- *Equality rights* – Some people, including some people of faith, believe that dementia is a form of affliction that a person has brought on themselves, or that dementia can be transmitted like an infectious disease. Both views can partly be understood when apocalyptic language describing dementia as a 'time bomb', 'living death' or an 'epidemic' are commonly used in the media and elsewhere. Yet both views are extremely unhelpful and no form of dementia is infectious. It is unclear what has really motivated the custodian at the temple to prohibit Hari from going there but they are discriminating against him on the grounds of disability and denying him his right to worship.

  Hari also has a right to confidentiality and respect for his private and family life. Providing he has mental capacity to make the decisions, it is he who decides who he discloses information to about his diagnosis. It is a breach of laws on privacy for the custodian to tell other members of the temple and shows little respect for Hari's private and family life.

- *Cognitive impairments as a disability* – It is not uncommon for people with Alzheimer's disease to 'time shift' back to an earlier phase of their life, and interpret the world around them and behave according to reference points from that time. Hari's reversion to speaking Punjabi may indicate that he believes he is much younger and is no longer able or willing to use English. The hostility he expresses towards the Muslim members of staff in the care home may reflect hostility he felt when he lived in India that existed between Sikh and Muslim communities across the border between India and Pakistan. It could be argued that it would be discriminatory to make Hari leave the care home and a denial of his social care rights if the home is inadequate in its response compared with other similar homes that could manage this. For example, his hostility could be addressed by trying to distract him from those beliefs and recruiting more Punjabi-speaking staff. However, if this is not possible, then for Hari's sake and the sake of staff it may be necessary to look for another home.

Mary

Mary is an 89-year-old Irish woman living in a care home. She was diagnosed with vascular dementia six years ago. Her husband is no longer alive and her children have moved back to Ireland. Mary needs a lot of personal care from staff in the home. She has a great deal of difficulty communicating and sometimes says she wants to 'go home', although she no longer has anywhere else to live. One member of staff always puts on an Irish accent when she speaks to Mary and describes Mary as 'daft'. Mary seems confused and upset when this happens, and keeps on asking the member of staff who she is. Staff members rarely ask Mary what she wants or ask Mary's permission to do things. Mary sometimes holds the hand of another female resident and staff had initially discouraged this but separating them caused both residents to become distressed so they decided to let them do it. When Mary's daughter phones the home she is told by the care home manager that staff make decisions for Mary 'because she has dementia' and she often tries to leave the home but they don't let her because 'she wouldn't be safe'. The daughter asks if the law allows them to do that. The manager says she doesn't know much about the law but that the home has its own rules to stop people like Mary leaving. When the manager describes Mary holding hands with another resident, her daughter becomes upset and says staff should separate them, saying 'It's not appropriate' and Mary's 'not like that.'

Commentary and key points

- *Right to protection from discrimination and abuse* – Mary is having her rights not to be discriminated against violated. She is being harassed on the grounds of nationality and race by the member of staff and therefore discriminated against. Because she has difficulty understanding and communicating, she is unable to ask the member of staff to refrain from speaking to her in the way they do. Mary is also the subject of discriminatory and emotional abuse from the member of staff because she is someone with care and support needs under the Care Act 2014 in England (previously referred to as 'vulnerable') so there is also a statutory safeguarding issue.

  The member of staff needs to be told to stop talking to Mary in that way and for the reasons to be explained. If this action is not taken, then the home itself could be accused of institutional abuse as it has not done anything to protect Mary's right not to be abused or discriminated against.

- *Decision making and deprivation of liberty* – Mary's rights under the MCA are not being respected because there is little evidence that staff are trying to help her make decisions on a decision-specific basis and there is the blanket assumption she cannot make decisions because of her dementia. However, staff do respect Mary's wish to hold hands with another resident. There could be a number of reasons why she holds hands (e.g. need for affection or reassurance, belief that she's a relative, attraction to women that her family were unaware of). Staff need to discuss these with Mary's daughter and how they may relate to dementia, as well as explain that the hand-holding seems to be something both residents want to do and brings them comfort and wellbeing. The daughter has the cognitive ability to understand this and recognise that it is the best interests of the person, not their relatives, that guide decisions.

  Mary, like many people with dementia in care homes, is not free to leave and does not have the mental capacity to consent to staying in the home. She also requires a lot of supervision. She is entitled to the legal safeguards of DoLS. It is not acceptable for a care home only to have its own rules for stopping people like Mary from leaving. Mary is entitled to have her rights protected under DoLS, which requires an application and authorisation process by the local authority – without it, Mary's human rights under Article 5 are being violated.

General commentary for all the scenarios

Cheryl, Hari and Mary all have rights as people with cognitive impairments caused by dementia under the articles of the UNCRPD. Examples of some of these rights can be found in Table 7.1. They include rights protecting their freedoms (e.g. right to life, liberty) but also rights of access to services and opportunities to enable their participation in society as equal citizens to people without disabilities (e.g. access to health services, employment opportunities, decision making, and choices regarding independent living). Under the UNCRPD, they also have the right to protection from discrimination in the way other relevant articles of the convention are applied.

Conclusion

It has been a slow journey bringing rights-based approaches, dementia, race and ethnicity together. It is also a complicated journey because of the intersectionality of multiple factors such as personal, family and community identity, disability and co-morbidities, lived experience and legal frameworks. Yet in the so-called 'age of austerity', where access to public services is becoming ever more restricted, causing the greatest difficulty to people who are often the most excluded, rights become ever more important. Awareness and understanding of rights can secure access to services and appropriate care, treatment and support. Rights-based approaches, including human rights-based approaches, are crucial in ensuring that policy and service development for people with dementia and their carers are legal, ethical and responsive to them, recognising their status in relation to disability and as citizens. A focus on rights and human rights in everyday practice in dementia care also enables a broader and more inclusive approach than a biomedical focus offers and can be both empowering and protective, as well as helpful for practitioners. It is vital that both the rights of people with dementia and people from BAME communities are explicitly recognised and there is a clear need for, and clear benefits to, applying them in unison. Rights, especially rights associated with equality, underpin person-centred dementia care, make it responsive to diverse populations and therefore enable it also to be truly citizen-centred.

Key messages

- Organisations representing, working with, or supporting BAME people with dementia and their families need to make ongoing efforts to raise awareness of the links between dementia, rights, equalities and human rights among individuals, families and organisations in BAME communities. As part of this awareness-raising, they need to support activism that enables the voice of people with dementia from BAME communities and their families to be heard.

- Organisations representing, working with, or supporting BAME people with dementia and their families need to be aware of, understand and respect how individuals wish to define themselves and this may not include identifying themselves as 'rights holders'. Organisations, however, need to have expertise available that can make the links between dementia, diversity and equalities, and relevant legal frameworks, including the UNCRPD. This should guide policy and practice but also be available, where necessary, to bring legal challenges on behalf of individuals.

- The development of policies, services and practice affecting all people with dementia should be based on or incorporate an explicit human-rights-based approach such as the PANEL principles, with the UNCRPD as its foundation. By using the PANEL principles there should be a clear focus on the involvement, experiences and needs of BAME people with dementia and their families, their rights to services, their decision making and their disability, equalities and human rights, as equal citizens of society.

References and links

Age UK (2011) *Older People and Human Rights: A Reference Guide for Professionals Working with Older People*. London: Age UK. Available at: www.ageuk.org.uk/Documents/EN-GB/For-professionals/Equality-and-human-rights/Older_People_Human_Rights__Expert_series_pro.pdf?dtrk=true [accessed 02/03/2018].

All Party Parliamentary Group on Dementia (2013) *Dementia does not discriminate: The experiences of black, Asian and minority ethnic communities*. London: All Party Parliamentary Group on Dementia. Available at: https://www.alzheimers.org.uk/download/downloads/id/1857/appg_2013_bame_report.pdf [accessed 11/03/2018].

Alzheimer Scotland (2009) *Charter of Rights for People with Dementia and their Carers*. Glasgow: Alzheimer Scotland. Available at: www.alzscot.org/assets/0000/2678/Charter_of_Rights.pdf [accessed 02/03/2018].

Alzheimer Scotland (n.d.) *Rights-based approaches to dementia.* Available at: www.alzscot. org/campaigning/rights_based_approach [accessed 02/03/2018].

Alzheimer's Society (2015) *Alzheimer's Society's view on equality, discrimination, and human rights.* London: Alzheimer's Society. Available at: www.alzheimers.org.uk/ info/20091/what_we_think/141/equality_discrimination_and_human_rights [accessed 02/03/2018].

Alzheimer's Society (2017) *List of Issues in Relation to the Initial Report of the United Kingdom of Great Britain and Northern Ireland* [In Relation to the CRPD]. Available at: www.alzheimers.org.uk/download/downloads/id/3631/submission_to_uncrpd_ committee_on_dementia.pdf [accessed 02/03/2018].

Blood, I. and Bamford, S. (2010) *Equality and Diversity and Older People with High Support Needs.* York: Joseph Rowntree Foundation. Available at: www.jrf.org.uk/sites/files/jrf/ supporting-older-people-full.pdf [accessed 02/03/2018].

Butchard, S. and Kinderman, P. (2017) 'Me and my life: Identity, human rights and dementia.' *Nursing Times*, 7/9/2017. Available at: www.nursingtimes.net/opinion/ expert-opinion/me-and-my-life-identity-human-rights-and-dementia/7021168.article [accessed 02/03/2018].

Curtice, M.J. and Exworthy, T. (2010) 'FREDA: A human rights-based approach to healthcare.' *The Psychiatrist*, 34, 150–156.

Dementia Alliance International (2016) *The Human Rights of People Living with Dementia: From Rhetoric to Reality.* Available at: www.dementiaallianceinternational.org/wp- content/uploads/2016/10/The-Human-Rights-of-People-Living-with-Dementia-from- Rhetoric-to-Reality_2nd-Edition_July-2016_English.pdf [accessed 02/03/2018].

Dementia Policy Think Tank, DEEP Network, Innovations in Dementia Community Interest Company (2017) *Our Lived Experience: Current Evidence on Dementia Rights in the UK. An Alternative Report to The UNCRPD Committee.* Available at: www.innovationsindementia.org.uk/wp-content/uploads/2018/01/Our-Lived- Experience-270717.pdf [accessed 08/02/2019].

Department of Health (2009) *Living Well with Dementia: A National Strategy.* Available at: www.gov.uk/government/uploads/system/uploads/attachment_data/file/168220/ dh_094051.pdf.

Department of Health (2014) *Care and Support Statutory Guidance.* London: Department of Health. Most recent version (updated 2018) available at: www.gov.uk/government/ publications/care-act-statutory-guidance/care-and-support-statutory-guidance.

Department of Health (2015) *Prime Minister's Challenge on Dementia 2020.* Available at: www.gov.uk/government/publications/prime-ministers-challenge-on-dementia-2020.

Gove, D.M., Andrews, J., Capstick, A., Geoghegan, C. *et al.* (2017) *Dementia as a Disability: Implications for Ethics, Policy and Practice. Ethical Discussion Paper.* Alzheimer Europe. Available at: www.alzheimer-europe.org/Ethics/Ethical-issues-in- practice/2017-Dementia-as-a-disability-Implications-for-ethics-policy-and-practice.

Hare, P. (2016) *Our Dementia, Our Rights.* The Dementia Policy Think Tank (part of the Dementia Engagement and Empowerment Project) and Innovations in Dementia Community Interest Company. Available at: http://dementiavoices.org.uk/wp-content/ uploads/2016/11/Our-dementia-Our-rights-booklet.pdf [accessed 02/03/2018].

HM Government (2010) *Equality Act 2010.* London: Stationery Office. Available at: www. legislation.gov.uk/ukpga/2010/15/pdfs/ukpga_20100015_en.pdf.

House of Lords (2014) *Mental Capacity Act 2005: Post-legislative scrutiny.* Select Committee on the Mental Capacity Act 2005 Report of Session 2013–14. London: The Stationery Office. Available at: https://publications.parliament.uk/pa/ld201314/ldselect/ldmentalcap/139/139.pdf [accessed 10/03/2018].

McGettrick, G. (2015) *Dementia, Rights and the Social Model of Disability.* London: Mental Health Foundation. Available at: www.mentalhealth.org.uk/sites/default/files/dementia-rights-policy-discussion.pdf [accessed 12/03/2018].

Mental Health Foundation (2008) *Engaging with Black and Minority Ethnic Communities about the Mental Capacity Act.* London: Mental Health Foundation.

Moriarty, J. and Manthorpe, J. (2012) *Diversity in Older People and Access to Services – An Evidence Review.* London: Age UK. Available at: www.ageuk.org.uk/globalassets/age-uk/documents/reports-and-publications/reports-and-briefings/equality-and-human-rights/rb_2012_equalities_evidence_review_moriarty.pdf [accessed 02/03/2018].

NHS Digital (2016) *Mental Capacity Act 2005, Deprivation of Liberty Safeguards (England) Annual Report 2015–16.* Available at: https://digital.nhs.uk/catalogue/PUB21814 [accessed 10/03/2018].

Oliver, M. and Sapey, B. (2012) *Social Work with Disabled People* (first edition published in 1983). Basingstoke: Palgrave Macmillan.

Scottish Government (2013) *Scotland's National Dementia Strategy 2013–2016.* Edinburgh: Scottish Government. Available at https://www2.gov.scot/Resource/0042/00423472.pdf [accessed 10/03/19].

Scottish Human Rights Commission (2009) *Human Rights in a Health Care Setting: Making it Work – An Evaluation of a Human Rights-Based Approach at The State Hospital, Glasgow.* Scottish Human Rights Commission. Available at: www.scottishhumanrights.com/media/1552/hrhcsfinalversion.pdf [accessed 02/03/2018].

Shakespeare, T., Zeilig, H. and Mittler, P. (2017) 'Rights in mind: Thinking differently about dementia and disability.' *Dementia,* 0, 0, 1–14. doi: 10.1177/1471301217701506.

The Guardian (2018) 'Londoner denied NHS cancer care: "It's like I'm being left to die".' Available at: www.theguardian.com/uk-news/2018/mar/10/denied-free-nhs-cancer-care-left-die-home-office-commonwealth [accessed 10/03/2018].

Truswell, D. (2018) 'Dementia, human rights and BAME communities.' *Journal of Dementia Care,* 28, 1, 22–23.

United Nations (2006) *United Nations Convention on the Rights of Person with Disabilities Optional Protocol* (Preamble). Available at: www.un.org/disabilities/documents/convention/convoptprot-e.pdf.

Voluntary Organisations Disability Group (2016) *Dementia: Equity and Rights.* London: Voluntary Organisations Disability Group. Available at: www.vodg.org.uk/wp-content/uploads/2016-VODG-Dementia-equity-and-rights-report.pdf [accessed 13/03/2018].

Watchman, K. (2016) *Dementia and Equality – Meeting the Challenge in Scotland.* Edinburgh: NHS Health Scotland. Available at: www.healthscotland.scot/media/1226/27797-dementia-and-equality_aug16_english.pdf [accessed 13/03/2018].

Williams, V., Boyle, G., Jepson, M., Swift, P., Williamson, T. and Heslop, P. (2014) 'Best interests decisions: Professional practice in health and social care.' *Health and Social Care in the Community*, 22, 1, 78–86.

Williamson, T. (2016) *Mapping Dementia Friendly Communities Across Europe*. Brussels: European Foundations' Initiative on Dementia. Available at: https://ec.europa.eu/eip/ageing/sites/eipaha/files/results_attachments/mapping_dfcs_across_europe_final.pdf [accessed 13/03/2018].

Table 7.1: Key UNCRPD articles for people with dementia

Article	Title	The right to (on an equal basis with non-disabled people)...
3	General principles	Respect for dignity and autonomy, non-discrimination, participation and inclusion, respect for differences, equality of opportunity, accessibility, gender equality
4	General obligations	General duties to promote the UNCRPD through legislation, practice, research, training, etc.
9	Accessibility	Access environments, transport, information, services
10	Right to life	Enjoy life on an equal basis with others
12	Equal recognition before the law	Enjoy legal capacity on an equal basis with others in all aspects of life.

Supported decision making that respects the person's, autonomy, will and preferences |
| 13 | Access to justice | Use of the judicial system |
| 14 | Liberty and security of person | Full legal protection if deprived of their liberty |
| 19 | Living independently and being included in the community

(Sections a, b, c) | Choose place of residence

Access to community support to live and remain in the community

Services for the general population which are inclusive of people with disabilities |
20	Personal mobility	The mobility support to be able
25	Health	Good health and health services
26	Habilitation and rehabilitation	Rehabilitation, reablement and support services
27	Work and employment	
28	Adequate standard of living and social protection	Comprehensive access to services, including work, adequate standard of living, participation in civic life, culture/recreation/sport
29	Participation in political and public life	
30	Participation in cultural life, recreation, leisure and sport	

CHAPTER 8

Exploring Spirituality and Dementia

David Truswell and Dr Natalie Tobert

Introduction

Increasing attention is being paid in the dementia literature (Agli, Bailly and Ferrand 2015) to the role that spirituality plays in the lives of those living with dementia, and their carers (Kaye 2000; Lawrence and Head 2005; Preston-De Vries 1998). However, the area still remains very much under-explored, with many commentators using a narrow concept of spirituality that focuses on mainstream US and European Christian ministry when considering how people living with dementia, and their carers, may benefit from spirituality as a supporting resource.

In this chapter, the authors propose that thinking about spirituality in dementia care and support should extend beyond institutional religion, encompassing individual perspectives that may be atheist, numinous, ecstatic, revelatory or existential. They also argue that often when spiritual needs are considered in the delivery of mainstream institutional care, this consideration is framed within a tradition of providing mainstream healthcare support and institutional forms of ministry that can fail to engage with the spiritual challenges that the person living with dementia, and their carers, may be experiencing.

The main forms of dementia that are the focus of this account are those often developing in later life, of which the most prevalent are Alzheimer's disease and vascular dementia. However, the account has general relevance across the experience of other forms of dementia.

Various meanings of spirituality

Sometimes spirituality might mean our ways of being in the world, our practices such as prayer, devotion or profound listening, our values such as compassion or integrity, or our feelings of relationship with others. Alternatively, it might mean our existential beliefs about being human or our understanding of the individual self and the person. It may also be understood as our actual human experiences, altered states of consciousness, or religious experiences (Tobert 2010a).

The issue is complex, for in addition to the variables of understanding 'spirituality' from a Eurocentric perspective, people have many cultural ways of understanding their health (Tobert 2010b). It is important for carers and those who experience dementia to have their cultural frameworks acknowledged. When there is a deeper understanding between mainstream service providers and their clients, together with an acknowledgement of different models of life, there may be a healing response shift.

Spirituality and dementia research

People living with dementia, and those close to them, are often shaken to their core by the diagnosis of dementia, and the sense of spiritual challenge that can arise frequently tests the foundations of any previous formal or informal 'faith' they may have had. In such circumstances, assessment of 'spiritual needs' has to be more nuanced than the simple identification of the person's adherence to particular 'tick box' categorisation of religion to be responded to by arranging sessions with a local priest, imam, rabbi or equivalent religious counsellor (Molly 2007; Van der Steen *et al.* 2014).

Religion is usually a practice or ritual within a community organisation, with worship, a set of sacred truths, and an agreed concept of divinity. Personal experience of spirituality may not fit neatly within a fixed religion. However, both may involve mystical experiences, which challenge a person's beliefs about the nature of reality and may involve a different route through society.

The authors challenge the common assumption made by dementia care professionals that those living with dementia, and their carers, who are from those cultural and ethnic groups referred to in the UK as Black, Asian and minority ethnic (BAME) communities have some long-standing traditional cultural expertise with dementia that includes a cultural recipe for dealing with the spiritual challenges of living with dementia.

Globally, dementia is the most challenging health economic issue of the 21st century (World Health Organization 2012). As a consequence of worldwide improvements in longevity, the rising incidence of Alzheimer's disease and vascular dementia – the most common forms of dementia affecting people in later life – accounts for an increasing proportion of health and social care spending in all societies.

The scale of the economic impact of dementia has been estimated globally at US $818 billion affecting an estimated 47 million people (Prince *et al.* 2016) worldwide. In the UK, there has been a substantial campaign to reduce the stigma faced by people living with dementia and create a more 'dementia-friendly' society, although it is recognised that these campaigns against stigma have not been very effective in their impact on BAME communities.

Campaigns may fail to have an impact on UK BAME communities as they are using Eurocentric strategies (Tobert 2010a). Also, there may be assumptions made about people who look ethnically the same, practise the same religion, and wear the same clothing, but have quite different personal narratives.

The ways we understand individual nationality are complex. For example, in the UK although legally this might be defined through census categories, there are many shades of understanding at a personal level. Being British may be seen as a matter of citizenship or being born in the UK. Narrow thinking might suggest that skin colour, religion or ethnicity are indicators of a personal sense of British nationality. Our skill in speaking English, eating the right food, having the appropriate clothing or the correct historical narratives (Tobert 2016) may have come to define a particular sense of Britishness in later life but have radically changed over the course of a lifetime. Dementia can return the individual to earlier ideas of the self and nationality.

There may be very different ways of understanding health both between and within communities. Subtle racism may exist unconsciously in our assumptions about our fellow human beings (Fernando 2014).

Side by side with the efforts to reduce stigma surrounding dementia, there has been a developing concern about the human rights of those living with dementia and also the rights of their family and carers.

However, much of the emphasis for investment in research on dementia and improvements in supporting those living with dementia is focused on developing a pharmacological treatment, with regular media articles misrepresenting the possibility of an imminent 'cure'.

A more sober consideration of the current state of thinking about the development of pharmacological treatments for dementia (Berk and Sabbagh 2013; Cummings, Morstor and Zhong 2014; Reitz 2012) and the scale of the problem in comparison with the scale of funding (Luengo-Fernandez, Leal and Gray 2015) would suggest that speculation about the state of development of a pharmaceutical solution should be treated with more caution (Mullane and Williams 2013). Older people with dementia live with multiple chronic health issues alongside their dementia, and a successful treatment, for example, of Alzheimer's disease alone will not have 100 per cent efficacy for all those with Alzheimer's. It may also have distressing side effects.

The authors favour an approach to supporting those living with dementia, and their family and carers, that is more explicit in its intention to do no harm.[1] From this perspective, the development of a social approach to supporting people living with dementia provides a more pragmatic model grounded in their daily experience. Considering spiritual needs in this context requires a deep focus on individual rights and the individual's understanding of themselves as they live through a profoundly challenging experience.

Individuality, spirituality and dementia

People living with dementia have mounted a strong challenge to the institutionalised and institutionalising categorisation of their personal situation that identifies them as 'service users' or 'sufferers' to counter their experience of social exclusion both from everyday life and from other users of health services (Swaffer 2016). In practice, until the symptoms of dementia become severe, those living with dementia often have limited access to health services, and any access they have is largely related to health issues other than their dementia.

Those living with dementia value the recognition of their individuality as they insist on and secure their inclusion in the everyday social world. This individuality should not be presumed to be static or assumed as only capable of being viewed as increasingly lost through the progress of the illness. People living with dementia also develop, either through continuing to pursue their previous developmental aspirations or through finding new aspirations through their experience of living with dementia. Spirituality has the potential to provide an anchor to individual identity and also to offer a supporting route to personal development. While for some these benefits may arise out of the assurance provided by the practices of a particular religion, for others the assurance may arise out of a more individualised approach to spiritual development.

---

1   http://breggin.com/special-topics/legal-page

In the early stages of the experience of dementia people may look for an explanation of their symptoms in terms of their personal faith. Among many non-European communities it is not uncommon to find explanations of dementia framed around folk traditions and beliefs (Garrett *et al.* 2015). These explanations can involve negative judgements of the person living with dementia or family members that can lead to both the person living with dementia, and family members, being isolated from their community. It is often assumed by health professionals in the UK that faith organisations within these communities will provide positive, spiritually led support for the person living with dementia, and their family, and also that the community will generally rally round to give support. This is rarely the case.

Furthermore, among some people, sickness is linked to ecological wrong-doing, or their dissatisfied or discarnate ancestors, but unless they feel their health professional is able to accept this, they may remain silent about their theories of illness causation (Tobert 2014).

There is also the potential for negative judgements about dementia found within faith narratives to have an unhelpful impact. However, in exploring the benefits of supporting spiritual needs, the potential negative impact of faith-based support could be regarded in the same way as the risk of harmful side effects in pharmacological interventions. The magical thinking that accompanies some mainstream interpretations of the results of current pharmacological research might also benefit from being subjected to more sceptical scrutiny (Moncrieff 2013).

It is not suggested that a spiritual perspective provides an easy panacea. Folk beliefs attributing the causes of dementia to spiritual factors can be a source of delay in access to treatment, as symptoms in the earlier stages are attributed to spiritual causes (Mukadam, Cooper and Livingston 2011; Uppal and Bonas 2014; Tobert 2010a). There is evidence that nursing staff are not comfortable working with spiritual beliefs that are unfamiliar to them (Skomakerstuen Ødbehr *et al.* 2015) and medical staff are reluctant to provide spiritual care at the end of life (Balboni 2014). Daly and Fahey-McCarthy (2014) argue that nurses and clinicians need to address this challenge from the wider perspective of spirituality rather than religious affiliation. Jolley and Moreland (2011) also argue persuasively for a personalised approach to high-quality nursing home care that includes a spiritual perspective. Approaches such as the Namaste programme (Sander 2014) offer a way of recognising individual spirituality throughout the illness into the very late stages of dementia. But such programmes lack the research investment that would better identify their benefits and support their development into mainstream care and support services.

While there are some initiatives supported by certain local faith communities working to raise dementia awareness and provide support directly through the congregation in the community, the challenge of reducing stigma remains substantial across all faiths. This includes the mainstream Christian ministries. There are individual stories from people living with dementia of their own personal journey of spiritual development through their faith while living with dementia, but healthcare professionals and dementia research take limited consideration of these accounts as a basis for enabling the preservation of identity, meaning and resilience by both those living with dementia, and their relatives and carers (Abu-Raiya and Pargament 2015; Douek 2015; Marquez-Gonzalez *et al.* 2012). Meeting spiritual needs could provide the support some people need to keep hold of their sense of themselves when other aspects of their lives and healthcare services cannot do this (Beuscher 2007; Downey 2009; Glueckauf *et al.* 2009).

It may feel as if society's advance in technology shifts the focus away from a caring model to one that is oriented towards technology and cure. Although technology may allow us the skills to increase our lifespan, physicians may still serve a person holistically and this is valued by patients (Koenig 2007; Puchalski 2001).

Therapeutic communication is important in compassionate care to negotiate with a patient and their carers, working within each framework of understanding. In the process of finding the most appropriate healing strategy, staff should acknowledge plural levels of understanding between clinician and patient.

Faith and spirituality as a personal resource in dementia

Often BAME communities in the UK are identified as providing negative and judgemental spiritual explanations of dementia. Yet across all faith communities there is limited consideration of dementia as a spiritual challenge. Individuals may view their experience of dementia, whether as a person living with dementia or caring for someone living with dementia, as a personal test of faith. Across all faiths, spiritual beliefs can be mobilised to support people living with dementia, and their carers (Meyer *et al.* 2015). The personal sense of a test of faith can be a challenge for an institutionalised perspective on spirituality, not only by care services but also by an institutionalised approach to ministry.

Fieldwork conducted by one of the authors with people of African and Indian origin showed that there were different but deep beliefs in supernatural causes of ill-health, including the effects of karma, the planets, reincarnation, the evil eye, and the ghosts of ancestral beings (Tobert 2016). Psychiatrists are becoming more interested in spiritual and cultural interpretations of symptoms, and the Royal College of Psychiatry has special interest groups (SIGs) reflecting this: one on trans-cultural psychiatry,[2] and another on spirituality.[3]

Some people believe that life is a cycle of birth, death and rebirth, so the spirit never dies, but is transformed. Although they understand that the physical body is no longer present, many feel they keep a relationship with the living and act as spiritual guardians.

A wider perspective on spirituality opens the door to looking at other ways of working with support for people living with dementia, for example 'mindfulness' (Robertson 2015), which may also be helpful for carers. While some accounts have explored spirituality as a resource in relation to BAME communities (Apesoa-Varano *et al.* 2015), it is seldom considered as a subject for consideration across the mainstream populations from any perspective other than Christianity (Ennis and Kazer 2013; Power 2006; Shealy McGee and Myers 2014).

A research study at Yale University investigated mental health clinicians' ontological beliefs about mental disorders. It explored clinicians' beliefs about biological, psychological, and environmental bases of disorders, and then investigated the consequences of their beliefs for judging effectiveness of treatment. Clinicians treated conditions differently: their beliefs had implications about effectiveness of psychotherapy or medication, and therefore their choice of treatment options for patients (Woo-kyoung, Proctor and Flanagan 2009).

More recently, there has been growing appreciation of the wider perspective on spirituality in dementia care. Anbäcken, Minemoto and Fujii 2015) illustrate powerfully the role that cultural expectations in Japan play in shaping the lives of those living with dementia, influencing perceptions of competence, self-determination and the sense of belonging. Johnson-Bogaerts (2015) draws

---

2   www.rcpsych.ac.uk/workinpsychiatry/specialinterestgroups/transculturalpsychiatry.aspx

3   www.rcpsych.ac.uk/workinpsychiatry/specialinterestgroups/spirituality.aspx

attention to the increasing importance of spirituality in palliative care across cultures and beliefs, using examples from Buddhist and Māori traditions. Hansenn (2013) highlights the value of 'yoik', a communal singing tradition of the Sami people of Scandinavia, as a reminiscence trigger for older members of the Sami community living with the later stages of dementia.

Looking at the comparison with other stigmatised health issues, there are rather different outcomes for people diagnosed with schizophrenia in other parts of the world when holistic perspectives, including spiritual approaches, have been considered. The World Health Organization claims almost two-thirds of patients with schizophrenia in Nigeria and India had better outcomes than the 37 per cent in the West (Barbato 1998; Haro *et al.* 2011). Since the 1980s, 'open dialogue' has become the key psychiatric practice in Finland, and evidence there shows that this approach reduces hospitalisation, use of medication and relapse when compared with usual treatment strategies (Seikkula 2006). Books such as *Cultural Perspectives on Mental Wellbeing* (Tobert 2016) provide a global resource for developing a deeper understanding reflecting cultural humility.

Some concluding reflections on dementia and spirituality

The severity of the challenge of dementia and the personal distress that the condition causes, with the attendant social and psychological impact on the person diagnosed with dementia and their family and carers, understandably drives a wish to see all this banished by a pharmacological miracle. Alzheimer's disease and vascular dementia are by far the most prevalent forms of dementia in later life, when many of those older people developing these illnesses often have multiple other health issues and may also be at a stage of spiritual reflection on their life.

Although dementia is a terminal illness, those with a dementia diagnosis will usually live for many years with the illness. The dementia policy framework internationally places an emphasis on living well with dementia and on care being provided in a way that is personal to the person receiving the care. For many people living with dementia, and their carers and families, the experience of dementia is something lived through every day as a personal and spiritual challenge.

The inclusion of a spiritual perspective in thinking about the care and support needs of people living with dementia, and their families and carers, can bring into immediate focus the individual quality of life of all those concerned. Potentially it taps into sources of personal and interpersonal resilience that may have been forgotten or not considered possible. It can provide an anchoring point for identity and memory that persists beyond some of the more evident losses in the later stages of the illness. It can also provide an anchoring point in both immediate personal relationships and relationships with the community.

Spirituality sits within the wider context of a lack of support in both research funding and the training of professionals for more social approaches to supporting people living with dementia, and their family and carers. While some areas for caution have been raised in this chapter, considering the individual spiritual needs of people living with dementia has far greater potential for significant impact on quality of life, understanding individual needs and facilitating individual rights than the current status of pharmacological intervention. Much of this seems to pursue a pharmacological panacea with a religious fervour not substantially supported by the evidence coming out of pharmacological clinical trials.

The testimony of individuals living with dementia indicates that for some people their sense of a personal test of faith can provide a sense of personal meaning through spiritual revelation or recognition, whether this reflects their commitment to a particular religious belief or some entirely personal spiritual viewpoint or a mixture of both.

While it needs to be respected that the exploration of a spiritual perspective may not be what some people living with dementia would want, currently such an exploration is not even on offer in most cases where people feel they might want it; and when it is offered, it is usually restricted to a limited offer of access to ministry. The authors propose that the offer to explore spiritual needs opens up the possibility of a new avenue in the discussion with the person living with dementia about their personal perspective on care and support and quality of life. This same avenue of discussion might be shared productively with family members and carers and be a place where people might also talk about other important and sensitive issues, such as loss, legacy and the end of life. These important elements of the personal narrative of those living with dementia need to be recognised as central elements in thinking about quality of life for people living with dementia, and their carers and family. These are also important areas of dementia care and support that need research and development funding.

References

Abu-Raiya, H. and Pargament, K.I. (2015) 'Religious coping among diverse religions: Commonalities and divergences.' *Psychology of Religion and Spirituality*, 7, 1, 24–33.

Agli, O., Bailly, N. and Ferrand, C. (2015) 'Spirituality and religion in older adults with dementia: A systematic review.' *International Psychogeriatrics*, 27, 5, 715–725.

Anbäcken, E-M., Minemoto, K. and Fujii, M. 'Expressions of identity and self in daily life at a group home for older persons with dementia in Japan.' *Care Management Journals*, 16, 2, 64–78.

Apesoa-Varano, E.C., Tang-Feldman, Y., Reinhard, S.C., Choula, R. and Young H.M. (2015) 'Multi-cultural caregiving and caregiver interventions: A look back and a call for future action.' *Journal of the American Society on Ageing*, 39, 4, 39–48.

Balboni, M.J., Sullivan, A., Enzinger, A.C., Epstein-Peterson Z.D. *et al.* (2014) 'Nurse and physician barriers to spiritual care provision at the end of life.' *Journal of Pain and Symptom Management*, 48, 3, 400–410.

Barbato, A. (1998) *Schizophrenia and Public Health*. Geneva: World Health Organization.

Berk, C. and Sabbagh, M. (2013) 'Successes and failures for drugs in late-stage development for Alzheimer's disease.' *Drugs & Aging*, 10, 783–792.

Beuscher, L.M. (2007) 'Exploring the Role of Spirituality in Coping with Early Stage Alzheimer's Disease.' ProQuest Dissertations and Theses; Hospital Premium Collection.

Cummings, J.L., Morstor, M. and Zhong, K. (2014) 'Alzheimer's disease drug-development pipeline: Few candidates, frequent failures.' *Alzheimer's Research & Therapy*, 6, 37–43.

Daly, L. and Fahey-McCarthy, E. (2014) 'Attending to the spiritual in dementia care nursing.' *British Journal of Nursing*, 23, 14, 787–791.

Douek, S. (2015) 'Faith and spirituality in older people – a Jewish perspective.' *Working with Older People*, 19, 3, 114–122.

Downey, B. (2009) 'Approaches to aging: A conversation with Nader Shabahangi.' *Aging Today*, 30, 4, 11–13.

Ennis, Jr. E.N. and Kazer, M.W. (2013) 'The role of spiritual nursing interventions on improved outcomes in older adults with dementia.' *Holistic Nursing Practice*, 27, 2, 106–113.

Fernando, S. (2014) *Mental Health Worldwide, Culture, Globalization and Development*. London: Palgrave Macmillan.

Garrett, M.D., Baldridge, D., Benson, W., Crowder, J. and Aldrich, N. (2015) 'Mental health disorders among an invisible minority: Depression and dementia among American Indian and Alaska Native elders.' Special Issue: White House Conference on Aging. *The Gerontologist*, 55, 2, 227–236.

Glueckauf, R.L., Davis, W.S., Allen, K., Chipi, P. *et al.* (2009) 'Integrative cognitive–behavioral and spiritual counseling for rural dementia caregivers with depression.' *Rehabilitation Psychology*, 54, 4, 449–461.

Hanssen, I. (2013) 'The influence of cultural background in intercultural dementia care: Exemplified by Sami patients Scandinavian.' *Journal of Caring Sciences*, 27, 231–237.

Haro, J.M., Edgell, E.T., Novick, D., Alonso, J., Kennedy, L. and Jones, P.B. (2011) *The British Journal of Psychiatry*, 199, 3, 194–201.

Johnson-Bogaerts, H. (2015) 'Spiritual care is integral to compassionate care.' *Kai Tiaki Nursing New Zealand*, 21, 10, 29.

Jolley, D. and Moreland, N. (2011) 'Dementia care: Spiritual and faith perspectives.' *Nursing & Residential Care*, 13, 8, 388–391.

Kaye, J. (2000) 'Spirituality and the Emotional and Physical Health of Black and White Southern Caregivers of Persons with Alzheimer's Disease and Other Dementias.' ProQuest Dissertations and Theses; Hospital Premium Collection.

Koenig, H. (2007) *Spirituality in Patient Care*. Philadelphia, PA: Templeton Press.

Lawrence, R.M. and Head, J.H. (2005) 'A time capsule for patients with dementia? Royal Society of Medicine (Great Britain).' *Journal of the Royal Society of Medicine*, 98, 3, 116–118.

Luengo-Fernandez, R., Leal, J. and Gray, A. (2015) 'UK research spend in 2008 and 2012: Comparing stroke, cancer, coronary heart disease and dementia.' *BMJ Open*, 5: e006648. doi:10.1136/bmjopen-2014-006648.

Marquez-Gonzalez, M., Lopez, J., Romero-Moreno, R. and Losada, A. (2012) 'Anger, spiritual meaning and support from the religious community in dementia caregiving.' *Journal of Religion and Health*, 51, 179–186.

Meyer, O.L., Nguyen, H.K., Dao, T.N., Vu, P., Arean, P. and Hinton, L. (2015) 'The sociocultural context of caregiving experiences for Vietnamese dementia family caregivers.' *Asian American Journal of Psychology*, 6, 3, 263–272.

Molly, P. (2007) 'Client-centred care for the person with dementia: The essential spiritual dimension.' *Whitireia Nursing Journal*, 14; Hospital Premium Collection, 19–25.

Moncrieff, J. (2013) *The Bitterest Pills: The Troubling Story of Antipsychotic Drugs*. London: Palgrave Macmillan

Mukadam, N., Cooper, C. and Livingston, G. (2011) 'A systematic review of ethnicity and pathways to care in dementia.' *International Journal of Geriatric Psychiatry*, 26, 12–20.

Mullane, K. and Williams, M. (2013) 'Alzheimer's therapeutics: Continued clinical failures question the validity of the amyloid hypothesis—but what lies beyond?' *Biochemical Pharmacology*, 85, 289–305.

Power, J. (2006) 'Religious and spiritual care.' *Nursing Older People*, 7, 24–27. Hospital Premium Collection.

Preston-De Vries, M.J. (1998) 'Spirituality of Caregiver Wives of Dementia Patients.' ProQuest Dissertations and Theses; Hospital Premium Collection.

Prince, M., Comas-Herrera, A., Knapp, M., Guerchet, M. and Karagiannidou, K. (2016) *World Alzheimer Report 2016: Improving healthcare for people living with dementia*. Alzheimer's Disease International.

Puchalski, C. (2001) 'The role of spirituality in health care.' *Proceedings of Baylor University Medical Centre*, 14, 4, 352–357.

Reitz, C. (2012) 'Alzheimer's disease and the Amyloid Cascade Hypothesis: A critical review. *International Journal of Alzheimer's Disease*, doi:10.1155/2012/369808.

Robertson, G. (2015) 'Spirituality and ageing – the role of mindfulness in supporting people with dementia to live well.' *Working with Older People*, 19, 3, 123–133.

Sander, R. (2014) 'The Namaste programme: Honouring the spirit within.' *Nursing and Residential Care*, 4, 222–224.

Seikkula, J., Aaltonen, J., Alakare, B., Haarakangas, K., Keränen, J. and Lehtinen, K. (2006) 'Five-year experience of first-episode nonaffective psychosis in open-dialogue approach: Treatment principles, follow-up outcomes, and two case studies.' *Psychotherapy Research*, 16, 2, 214–228.

Shealy McGee, J. and Myers, D. (2014) 'Sacred relationships, strengthened by community, can help people with mild or early-stage Alzheimer's.' *Journal of the American Society on Ageing*, 38, 1, 61–67.

Skomakerstuen Ødbehr, L., Kvigne, K., Hauge, S. and Danbolt, L.J. (2015) 'A qualitative study of nurses' attitudes towards and accommodations of patients' expressions of religiosity and faith in dementia care.' *Journal of Advanced Nursing*, 71, 2, 359–369.

Swaffer, K. (2016) *What the Hell Happened to My Brain?: Living Beyond Dementia*. London: Jessica Kingsley Publishers.

Tobert, N. (2010a) *Bridging Cultures, Dissolving Barriers, Mental Health Promotion with BME Communities, End of Year Evaluation Report*. Harrow: NHS Harrow.

Tobert, N. (2010b) *Somali Advocacy Research Report*. Harrow: Mind in Harrow/Kings Fund.

Tobert, N. (2014) *Spiritual Psychiatries: Mental Health Practices in India and UK*. CreateSpace.

Tobert, N. (2016) *Cultural Perspectives of Mental Wellbeing*. London: Jessica Kingsley Publishers.

Uppal, G. and Bonas, S. (2014) 'Constructions of dementia in the South Asian community: A systematic literature review.' *Mental Health, Religion & Culture*, 17, 2, 143–160.

Van der Steen, J., Gijsbert, M-J., Hertogh, C. and Deliens, L. (2014) 'Predictors of spiritual care provision for patients with dementia at the end of life as perceived by physicians: A prospective study.' *BMC Palliative Care*, 13, 61.

Woo-kyoung, A., Proctor, C. and Flanagan, E. (2009) 'Mental health clinicians' beliefs about biological, psychological, and environmental bases of mental disorders.' *Cognitive Science*, 33, 2, 147–182.

World Health Organization (2012) *Dementia: A public health priority*. Geneva: World Health Organization.

CHAPTER 9

Dementia and Further Common Issues Affecting Several BAME Communities

David Truswell

Interpreting and translation

First-generation migrants to the UK will usually have grown up outside the UK speaking a language other than English, and however fluent and accomplished in English they later become, they may revert entirely to their mother tongue with the onset of dementia. Interpreting when working with families and people living with dementia has additional challenges to the already testing demands of interpreting in clinical settings. There has been very little attention paid to the complexities of interpreting in dementia care, exceptions being the work of Botsford and Harrison-Dening (2015) and Truswell and Tavera (2016)

One must turn to the US to find more extensive work on the role of interpreting in clinical/medical settings, although this is primarily focused on acute care. The general finding from this research is that professionally trained interpreters provide better outcomes and reduce non-compliance risk (Karliner *et al.* 2007). However, clinicians are often faced with strong family pressure to use family members as interpreters, who may withhold material from the patient or the clinician, or misreport for cultural reasons; or the clinician's advice and instruction to the patient may be misrepresented due to unfamiliarity. Many UK NHS trusts require clinicians to use professional interpreters in clinical consultations in preference to family or friends where possible. With cost pressures on NHS budgets pushing clinicians to make more use of telephone interpreting, dementia is one area where this may not be advisable as both the technical task and psychological dynamics of the situation are invariably more complex than in other clinical settings. Some of these complexities are illustrated in the following accounts.

The view of an interpreting agency

Beverley Costa was CEO of Mothertongue, a UK interpreting agency that specialisies in interpreting in mental health settings. Speaking to the author about her experience as a supervisor of interpreters working in dementia care settings, she made the following observations:

- The interpreter can find themselves in a confusing situation if the person living with dementia has some paranoid elements where they believe the people around them are conspiring against them or imagining conversations. In one example, a person who had been held captive in Russia during her earliest years imagined that those around her were speaking in Russian when they were speaking in English. The clinical staff had called in a Russian interpreter.

- Trust building by the interpreter with the person, family and also the clinical professionals is essential. The person living with dementia may prefer a family member to act as the interpreter, while clinicians may feel they need a professional interpreter for clinically safe interpreting. Interpreters will be under strong pressure from the family to be more of an advocate and befriender as the family may feel more helpless than in other clinical interpreting situations. The family can put the clinician under strong pressure to use family members as interpreters, and clinicians need to be sensitive in resisting. A balance between the use of family members and professional interpreters may need to be determined by the clinician on a case-by-case basis.

- Clinicians should have training in working with interpreters.

- Clinicians should assume that the case will be complex from the outset as there will be cultural issues the clinician is not aware of that the interpreter may be able to advise on, as well as language issues.

- When people living with dementia have lost their previously acquired language, they do not simply revert entirely to their previous language, as some elements of English or other languages learned later in life may be preserved as untranslatable neologisms.

- People may have grown up speaking local dialects involving terms or phrases that have fallen out of use or are not known to a contemporary interpreter and the interpreter may themselves be working with phrases and allusions in the language that are no longer in common use.

Kamaljit: An interpreter's story

Kamajit has been working as a professional interpreter for about ten years, with a number of interpreting sessions over that period taking place in the local memory clinic. She interprets for speakers of South Asian languages. She has worked both with people who have temporarily lost the use of English through a stroke and those with progressive loss through dementia. One thing that seems to happen with dementia is that the language gets much simpler and almost childlike; it can become repetitive or the speaker can become like an argumentative child.

A number of the older people she works with come from a rural part of India where they had their own dialect that they had spoken. They might teach their children to speak the local 'official' language for school but continue to speak between themselves in the local dialect. This can mean that if they develop dementia in later life and return to using the language of their own childhood, their children, who have lost fluency with the dialect, can't communicate with them.

As an interpreter, she feels she is under more pressure in these sessions to be a befriender. She can see and sense things that she knows are culturally important and that may not be coming across in the language, and the clinician probably does not notice while the patient may be struggling to put things into words. As an interpreter, she is not supposed to prompt people when they are trying to find words that are 'on the tip of their tongue'. These situations can be more like the kind of thing that happens with people with severe mental health problems. People can get very distraught and emotional, sometimes screaming and shouting, but it's more likely that they are stuck and become argumentative like a child would be, wanting something to be done their way.

Kamajit has worked with families both in the clinic setting and when they are interviewed at home, and it can be difficult. The families often don't feel they know what's happening and that the personality of the person living with dementia has changed. People in the Indo-Pakistani families she works with want to look after their parents at home, but they feel they are not appreciated. There may also be cultural issues that they don't speak about and she will pick these up. They will say to her that they feel she understands and turn to her to tell them what to do. But that is not her role as an interpreter. She wants to help them – that is why she became an interpreter – but she can't provide what they want as an interpreter.

She might have to ask the patient how they are being treated by the family and she must be very discreet in how she does this. The patient may say they are unhappy with the care and want to go home, but they often mean going home to India, which isn't possible. Alternatively, the patient may say they would prefer to be with other family members, and the family member who is caring for them feels they are not valued. None of this means that the patient is not getting good care, but how are these family members going to feel being told the patient feels care would be better somewhere else?

Sanmaya: An interpreter's story

Sanmaya is a Nepalese interpreter who has been working with memory services since 2010 as an interpreter, and before that for two years as a voluntary interpreter. She has interpreted for people living with dementia in a variety of settings, including memory clinics, GP surgeries and a local mental health hospital.

Interpreting in settings with people living with dementia is different from working in other interpreting settings. She has particularly noticed in assessments that about 50 per cent of what is happening is pointless. Most of the patients she is acting as the interpreter for have been brought up in very rural parts of Nepal and will have had no education. In the time and place they grew up, only people in the highest two castes would have been allowed to go to school. Asking them things like the time or to count backwards when they do not have any basic education makes no sense. Even when they ask people to copy a drawing, a lot of women from that background would never have held a pencil in their life – it's something women would not be allowed to do. When the patients are asked what month it is, Sanmaya has to work it out, which takes a bit of time because there is a different calendar in Nepal and the patients use the old Nepalese calendar, which she doesn't use anymore herself. Every time Sanmaya works with a new clinician, she must explain why it's taking her so long to translate the response. Another thing patients get asked is if they know what season it is. She doesn't think the clinician understands that where the patient grew up there are six seasons, and as they never attended school they would be unlikely to know the official season names. The seasons here are completely different. At one of her sessions in the hospital Sanmaya had to tell the clinicians what kind of questions to ask to find out more about the patient's memory.

She feels that people in the UK, one of the most technologically advanced countries in the world, may not visualise what a very under-developed country is like. The patients she is interpreting for come from an area that is more likely to resemble the 10th or

11th century. The country is mountainous and while things have got a bit better now, when the patients that she sees were growing up there would have been hardly any roads and people stayed were they were. They had local languages and dialects that they spoke. Nepalese would be a second language for them so when she interprets there are words she doesn't know from that local language that she herself has to guess at or work out. For her, the assessment can't be 100 per cent accurate because of these shortcomings. She feels that they should ask different questions, not always the same ones, which often don't make sense to the patients anyway.

Dementia, interpreting and translation

Many of the cohort of first-generation migrants arriving in the UK in early adulthood in the late 1950s or 1960s, and now likely to find themselves in dementia services, work in low-level jobs and do not have a basic level of education. They may be unable to read or write in their own native language, or speak languages that have no word for dementia or only derogatory terms. Written material in their mother tongue, either for the purpose of information on dementia or to evoke reminiscence, may have little value for them. The bulk of leaflets on dementia in translation must be set aside in favour of something more nuanced.

Interpreting in the clinical setting with someone who is living with dementia is more challenging than in other medical settings. Clinicians need to be trained to work effectively with professional interpreters, and both interpreters and clinicians will need to work to build the trust of patient and family in the interpreter's role as well as an understanding of its limits. The interpreter can help the clinician understand cultural cues, but these cues may only be visible in a physical meeting, not in telephone exchanges. Language changes over time, as does language use within families – children may literally not speak the same language as their parents, and a younger interpreter brought up in an urban culture may struggle with a form of the language used 60 years ago in an isolated rural community. Interpreters may need to familarise themselves with the vocabulary of dementia services before they can comfortably find a translatable equivalent for all the terms. Clinicians should build in time with the interpreter both pre- and post-assessment to ensure the interpreter understands what is happening and the clinician is fully debriefed.

The financial impact of dementia

Studies demonstrating the national economic cost of dementia (Prince *et al.* 2014) are commonplace in media headlines but less well explored is the economic cost to individual families and the more direct personal financial implications of living with dementia. Memory problems affect the ability to manage everyday cash transactions and, in the 21st-century digital society, have an impact on recall of PIN numbers, passwords and a host of digital security measures associated with routine financial transactions. We are all encouraged not to share these details with others. People living with dementia may also become suspicious that money or other assets are being stolen. First-generation migrants may have financial resources or assets located outside the UK, often linked to an aspiration to retire to their country of origin. Without allocating lasting power of attorney while they still retain the recognised mental capacity to do so, many people living with dementia risk getting into serious financial difficulty as the illness progresses. They may have no opportunity to make their own decisions on allocating a trusted individual to manage their property and financial affairs once they are deemed to lack mental capacity.

In the UK, there are two types of lasting power of attorney,[1] one for financial decisions and one for health and care. The former is the focus here, but one individual can be allocated to cover both financial affairs and health and care issues. Also, lasting power of attorney can be granted to more than one person to manage either an individual's financial affairs or their health and social care needs. The nominated person must be over 18 but does not have to live in the UK or be a UK citizen. This latter is significant for BAME communities.

People from BAME communities may be particularly financially vulnerable in later life (Khan 2008). For first-generation migrants, it is quite likely that their lifetime income has been low relative to the host country's majority population and that their level of pension entitlements will be low consequently (Khan and Mawhinney 2010). Demographically, the percentage of people from BAME communities who are homeowners is lower than the percentage of White UK nationals (Khan 2012). For those who own their homes, the home may be their single main financial asset, and the first-generation migrants may also own a home, or plot of land on which they intend to build a home, outside the UK. In the UK, these financial assets

---

1   www.gov.uk/power-of-attorney

will be taken into consideration in assessing their ability to pay for social care provision. Individuals would be best served by reviewing their financial planning as soon as possible if they are diagnosed with dementia so that they are able to make choices fully reflecting their own wishes and capacity.

For younger people living with dementia, there is the direct loss of income through increased absence from work due to illness, or the loss of employment. There is some evidence that younger onset dementia has a higher incidence in the UK African-Caribbean community (Adelman *et al.* 2011) but no studies examine if there is any disproportionate loss of employment of people from this community as a result of their dementia diagnosis.

Unpaid care accounts for 44 per cent of the costs of dementia in the UK (Prince *et al.* 2014), £11 billion of an estimated £26.3 billion. The methodology for the report that derives these costs refers to differential costs arising from the severity of the illness (Prince *et al.* 2014) and it would be useful to examine if, as a result of family carers from BAME communities providing family support for people who are more ill with dementia because of the pattern of delayed access to diagnosis, they incur more personal costs.

Some of the work done on racial differences in the risk of dementia in the US may be useful as a starting point for considering this. Yeo and Gallagher-Thompson's 2006 book of collected papers on the impact of dementia on US minority communities, *Ethnicity and the Dementias,* and a later 2014 literature review by Lines and Wiener (2014) identify the African-American and Caribbean Hispanic populations as having higher dementia rates than the US White majority. In a 2013 report, Gaskin, LaVeist and Richard comprehensively examine costs for the African-American community and estimate that 60 per cent of the $71.6 billion cost of caring for those in the African-American community living with dementia in 2012 was paid for by African-American families, of which $544 million was direct out-of-pocket expenses paid by the families.

The UK's Policy Research Institute on Ageing and Ethnicity (PRIAE), in a report (Patel 1999) on care services for BAME elders to the Royal Commission on Long Term Care, points out shortcomings in 'basic ordinary daily care requirements such as physical care, food, and ability to exercise religious/spiritual beliefs and communication' (p.269) for BAME elders. Today, PRIAE no longer exists. It is these insufficiencies in daily care requirements that we can expect to be a significant and routine supplementary cost for BAME families supporting relatives either in the community or in mainstream care facilities.

The author has heard several accounts by relatives of people living with dementia in BAME families of them purchasing additional culturally appropriate materials or support for those they are caring for who are living with dementia, either in the community or in residential care. This can include regularly purchasing food or cooked meals that are more culturally appropriate, regularly purchasing newspapers and magazines in languages other than English, and regularly paying for more appropriate grooming arrangements or personal care materials.

A consequence of the later presentation to diagnostic services by those who are living with dementia in BAME communities may be that it is too late for the individual living with dementia to be able to nominate lasting power of attorney as they may be found to lack sufficient mental capacity. It is not uncommon that spouses or children who have been acting as carers assume that they can automatically access and manage the financial affairs of the person living with dementia who has lost the capacity to manage this themselves, only to find this assumption is mistaken and they cannot simply pay bills, access bank accounts or sort out debt notifications on their behalf. Once the person has been identified as lacking capacity, the management of their financial affairs may involve application to the Court of Protection to appoint a deputy.

Culture Dementia UK,[2] an organisation that has done extensive work in raising awareness about dementia in BAME communities, places strong emphasis on promoting lasting power of attorney at its events, based on years of experience in advising and supporting BAME families who have had substantial financial difficulties while supporting someone living with dementia. The organisation also advocates that people do this through the relatively low-cost online application and registration as early as possible.

An estimated 61.3 per cent of people living with late onset dementia are living in the community.[3] For those living with dementia in the community it has been estimated that unpaid care meets 74.9 per cent of the costs (Prince *et al.* 2014).

Key unexamined questions for the cost of dementia to families in BAME communities are:

---

2   www.culturedementiauk.org

3   www.dementiastatistics.org/statistics/care-services

1. Does the necessity of paying routine additional costs for food, physical care needs and communication not provided by the mainstream services constitute a significant and unrecognised supplementary cost for dementia care in the BAME community?

2. Does caring for a family member in the community lead to more unpaid provision of higher value care by BAME families, involving both higher levels of direct input in respect of hours of care provided or levels of severity managed? If so, what are the economic consequences? What are the implications for the training and support needs of BAME carers in these circumstances?

There should be an examination of these possible cost disparities to BAME families to ensure that the families do not continue to financially supplement the care system's failure to cover institutionalised shortfalls in equitable provision of dementia care.

The risk of elder abuse

In other chapters of this book, authors critically examine the view that people in BAME communities can be assumed to 'look after their own' when supporting those living with dementia, but the issue of elder abuse in BAME communities is little examined or understood. The experience of dementia is a profound social and psychological challenge for the person living with dementia, and those with close relationships to them. Apart from cultural stigma regarding dementia, which has been identified by several authors, for many migrating families in the past 50 years this has also been a period where people live significantly longer, family size has reduced across migrant families to more resemble host community norms and contemporary families are more geographically dispersed. Family resources for care and support may well be substantially reduced because of migration, with the complex and long-term demands of supporting someone living with dementia severely challenging or sometimes exhausting these resources.

Individual family dynamics and culturally held expectations may lead family-based caring, particularly those providing the most time-consuming and challenging aspects of care, to be authoritatively delegated to the person in the family with the least influence on family decisions (Mohammed 2017), often reflecting gendered expectations of caring roles within the family (Parveen and Oyebode 2017). People may feel a sense of obligation or duty to act as carers (Parveen, Morrison and Robinson 2012) that exceeds their resources either due to lack of time or lack of psychological resources because of other demands. Issues of social standing or 'face' may lead to family carers becoming or feeling isolated from support from their own communities and wary of communicating feelings of helplessness, inadequacy and ignorance either within their own community or to 'outsiders' that may lead to community ostracism and potentially the lifelong label of being a 'bad' son or daughter.

Negative cultural stereotypes about dementia can be carried into the care setting by paid carers from the same cultural background as the person who is living with the dementia, leading to significant problems. This can include assuming the person who is living with dementia should not be allowed choices, assuming communications from the person living with dementia can be disregarded as they are 'crazy talk' or that the paid carer holds the defining view on what is culturally appropriate for the person they are caring for. This can mean, in some cases, poor care from paid carers from the same cultural background as the person living with dementia that may be difficult to challenge (Janet Jadavji, a BAME carer, personal communication, November 2018).

Aside from the cultural traditions of family caring, people may have poor relationships with other family members that will only sour further if they are obliged as a result of family pressure to care for these family members. A discussion on the balance between the emotional fulfilment and personal limits of carers and the needs of those living with dementia should be opened up across all communities. Media stories framed around 'battling' with dementia do no justice to the often devastating and painful realignments that dementia brings to the most intimate and long-standing relationships, as for example is illustrated by Wendy Williams in a blogpost recounting the changing relationship with her daughters.[4]

Truswell and Hinds (2018) argue that the relationship between the carer and person who is living with dementia should be viewed from an 'emotional intelligence' perspective that acknowledges and equally respects the needs and wishes of both the carer and the person living with dementia. There are some reports that suggest that where cultural traditions of community support have been mobilised to assist those families in the community supporting people living with dementia, this can be a benefit.

---

4   https://whichmeamitoday.wordpress.com/blog

The concept that BAME communities 'look after their own' leaves unexamined the possibility of an increased risk of elder abuse in what may be quite isolated families struggling to cope with an illness they barely feel able to understand, while at the same time feeling alienated from any of the respite or resilience that might be offered by their communities with other illnesses that do not carry the same stigma as dementia. The assumption that 'cultural matching' of care staff automatically produces culturally appropriate dementia care also needs to be challenged.

These unexamined assumptions increase the risk that poor or uninformed care, which may well be the result of lack of understanding and people simply getting out of their depth in a situation more psychologically challenging than they had realised, becomes entrenched as secretive abuse. The unsupported carers may become more isolated and embittered by the demands of providing care that they are psychologically unable to cope with. The spectrum of elder abuse and neglect is a complex area that does not only result from willful and malicious intent with clear intention to harm. It can also involve misunderstanding of the rights and capacities of those living with dementia in a way that leads to coercive controls and behavioural restrictions, for example locking older people with dementia in the house for fear of them wandering. The complexity of the risks of elder abuse in dementia need to be more robustly examined and understood. This is not solely an issue for BAME communities. Neglect of the issue of risk of elder abuse for those communities that it is assumed 'look after their own' should not be accepted.

Lack of appropriate reminiscence materials

There have been some remarkable developments in recent years with digitally based or 'virtual reality' materials in the UK for those of a majority White UK background living with dementia, such as collating audio materials (usually music) and visual materials including photographs, film or reconstructed scenes from a particular era.[5] While much of this material still awaits detailed evaluation, anecdotally the materials often generate improved engagement with people living with dementia, including those who may have withdrawn from socialising. Often the materials will provide an opportunity for sharing and discussing experiences in a group setting.

---

5   https://thewaybackvr.com

There is far less exploration of developing reminiscence materials for those living with dementia from BAME communities where first-generation migrants will have spent their early childhood outside the UK and materials that coincide with their point of arrival in the UK may also evoke memories of hostility and racism experienced at that time. The Pearl Support Network[6] is an organisation that has produced materials for use by the African-Caribbean community and is developing a web-based reminiscence tool utilising imagery and items that would be very familiar for people who emigrated to the UK from the Caribbean during the 1950s and 1960s. It has also developed reminiscence cue sheets and cards involving pictures of familiar objects for those growing up in the African-Caribbean community of the post-war era.

Residential and day services should be aware that while some of those using their services may respond and engage with reminiscence materials that are intended to evoke a particular historical era in the UK, there will be BAME people for whom the material has no relevance or may evoke negative memories. The challenge for developing a more person-centred approach to reminiscence that incorporates different cultural histories is how to best manage the materials used and gain more information on materials that can be used with those of BAME origin. There can potentially be a more enriching engagement for all through finding out about personal life histories that encompass a diversity in personal reminiscence across a variety of cultures.

A useful cautionary note on digital reminiscence resources is raised by Campt (2012) when looking at the use of archival photography within the African diaspora in Europe. In her meditation on the relationship between personal photographs and memory, she draws attention to the emotional significance of physically holding photographs and passing them around to talk about with others as resonating powerfully with the same acts of holding the photographs and discussing them with other family members or friends in the distant past. At the time when some migrants would have lived in circumstances without reliable access to electricity and were unlikely to have a TV, sharing photographs would have been a significant family social event. Scanning a photograph and displaying it on a screen does not have the same emotional resonance, but physically reproducing photographs that can be held and shared could well be more emotionally powerful.

A further cautionary note regarding stock photography and imagery from the past is that stock characters and advertising materials may include

---

6   https://pearlsupportnetwork.org.uk

representations of people from BAME communities that would be regarded as unacceptable and derogatory now, even if they were commonplace at the time. Services need to give this due consideration when selecting reminiscence materials for general use. Stock images may also present a stereotyped picture of particular aspects of history that excludes representation of the diversity that would have been current at the time, for example the frequent absence of Black or Asian soldiers in stock images representing those fighting in World War II, or the frequent absence of Black or Asian doctors or nurses in the pictorial portrayal of the early days of the NHS.

End-of-life care

End-of-life care in dementia has generally received limited attention and the needs of those from BME communities are barely explored in the UK apart from isolated work such as Calanzani, Koffman and Higginson's excellent 2013 review *Palliative and End of Life Care for Black, Asian and Minority Ethnic Groups in the UK*. Although the review does not have a focus on dementia, its main conclusion is highly material: '…a structured, coordinated national strategy is needed. This should be done as part of a strategy to provide the best palliative and end of life care possible for all, regardless of their ethnicity' (2013, p.50). This same continues to hold in 2018 (Koffman 2018).

Considerations in the literature or recent seminars on the role of faith in dementia support do not necessarily include an in-depth examination of the experience of end-of-life care, often focusing on the earlier stages rather than later stages of dementia when both the physical and mental capacity of those living with dementia may be very diminished.

People from BAME communities do not necessarily profess the Christian faith and those that do may belong to congregations practising Christian worship in a markedly different way to the traditional UK Church of England or Roman Catholic Church. It is gradually becoming more acknowledged that those in roles of religious ministry across all faiths need more education about dementia, although there is little research done on the stigma and stereotypes about dementia that may exist within the various faith institutions.

Shahid Mohammed in his 2017 account of caring for his mother while she was living with dementia gives a detailed and moving account of the good practice of his local services in supporting him through his mother's final days and respecting the values of his faith through the process. For many of those from BAME communities, funeral arrangements may be intensive and far-reaching family events involving mourning periods lasting several days, specific rituals having to be completed prior to or shortly after death, particular forms of burial or particular family members being expected to lead the organising of the funeral arrangements. If family members are located overseas, they may be expected to attend the funeral and any related ceremonies. As people from BAME communities living with dementia may tend to present to dementia diagnosis and support services later in the course of their illness, mental capacity concerns may complicate issues such as leaving a will or making agreements regarding disposal of assets, advanced directives, power of attorney and financial provision for the funeral. Planning for end-of-life care can be inhibited by issues such as cultural stigma about dementia, institutional mistrust of the medical services on the part of family carers, lack of cultural understanding by the medical service, and cultural norms regarding sharing information about impending death with the terminally ill.

Difficult though the conversations will be, the conversation about end-of-life care in some measure should begin as early as possible rather than be delayed until the last few weeks or days of life. A considerable amount of work needs to be done across all faiths and care providers to build both the skills and confidence of faith practitioners and service practitioners to support this. One should be mindful that those living with dementia with no professed faith may also have preferences for their end-of-life and funeral arrangements that should be explored at the point where they still have capacity to make choices in the matter.

References

Adelman, S., Blanchard, M., Rait, G., Leavey, G., and Livingston, G. (2011) 'Prevalence of dementia in African-Caribbean compared with UK-born White older people: Two-stage cross-sectional study.' *British Journal of Psychiatry*, 199, 2,119–125.

Botsford, J. and Harrison Dening, K. (2015) 'Working with interpreters in a dementia care setting.' *The Journal of Dementia Care*, 23, 6, 18–19.

Calanzani, N., Koffman, J. and Higginson, J. (2013) *Palliative and End of Life Care for Black, Asian and Minority Ethnic Groups in the UK.* London: Marie Curie Cancer Care.

Campt, T. (2012) *Image Matters; Archive, Photography and the African Diaspora in Europe.* Durham, NC: Duke University Press.

Gaskin, D., LaVeist, T. and Richard, P. (2013) *The Costs of Alzheimer's and Other Dementia for African Americans.* African American Network Against Alzheimer's.

Karliner, L.S., Jacobs, E.A., Chen, A.H. and Mutha, S. (2007) 'Do professional interpreters improve clinical care for patients with limited English proficiency? A systematic review of the literature.' *Health Services Research*, 42, 2, 727–754.

Khan, O. (2008) *Financial Inclusion and Ethnicity: An Agenda for Research and Policy Action*. London: Runnymede Trust.

Khan, O. (2012) *A Sense of Place: Retirement Decisions Among Older Black and Minority Ethnic People*. London: Runnymede Trust.

Khan, O. and Mawhinney, P. (2010) *The Costs of 'Returning Home': Retirement Migration and Financial Inclusion*. London: Runnymede Trust.

Koffman, J. (2018) *Dementia and End of Life Care for Black, Asian and Minority Ethnic Communities*. Better Health Briefing Paper 45. London: Race Equality Foundation.

Lines, L. and Wiener, J. (2014) *Racial and Ethnic Disparities in Alzheimer's Disease: A Literature Review*. Washington, DC: US Department of Health and Human Services.

Mohammed, S. (2017) *A Fragmented Pathway; Experiences of the South Asian Community and the Dementia Care Pathway: A Care Giver's Journey*. Salford: University of Salford.

Parveen, S., Morrison, V. and Robinson, C.A. (2012) 'Ethnicity, familism and willingness to care: Important influences on caregiver mood?' *Aging and Mental Health*, 17, 115–124.

Parveen, S. and Oyebode, J. (2018) *Dementia and Minority Ethnic Carers*. Better Health Briefing Paper 46. London: Race Equality Foundation.

Patel, N. (1999) 'Black and Minority Ethnic Elderly: Perspectives on Long-Term Care.' In *With Respect to Old Age: Long Term Care – Rights and Responsibilities* Report by the Royal Commission. London: Stationery Office.

Prince, M., Knapp, M., Guerchet, M., McCrone, P. *et al.* (2014) *Dementia UK: Update*. London: Alzheimer's Society.

Truswell, D. and Hinds, J.A. (2018) 'Emotional intelligence – helping carers to achieve balance.' *Journal of Dementia Care*, 26, 4, 28–29.

Truswell, D. and Tavera, Y. (2016) *An Electronic Resource Handbook for CNWL Memory Services: Dementia Information for Black, Asian and Minority Ethnic Communities*. London: Central and North West London NHS Foundation Trust. Available at: www.cnwl.nhs.uk/wp-content/uploads/Memory-Services-Handbook-final.pdf.

Yeo, G. and Gallagher-Thompson, D. (2006) *Ethnicity and the Dementias* (third edition). Abingdon, Oxford: Routledge.

CHAPTER 10

A Single Carer's Perspective of Dementia

Dr Shibley Rahman

Introduction

'Once you've met one person with dementia, you've met one person with dementia.' This phrase frequently and conveniently comes up at conferences on dementia, with invariably the same speakers, including the same academics, same person living with dementia, same carer, same charity representative and same policy lead. But it is little appreciated that *'Once you've met one carer of a person with dementia, you've met one carer of a person with dementia.'*

By virtue of this, you may agree with little, some, much or all of what I am about to say.

My mum lives with dementia. I live with my mum in a small flat in North London. I am a trained physician, and even then it wasn't obvious to me that my own mother was developing a dementia. Of course, doctors are told by their regulator not to involve themselves in the clinical care of family members.

My mum and I represent a difficult scenario, but not an altogether uncommon one. That is, of an unpaid carer who has a professional background in dementia. I am a member of the Royal College of Physicians of London, and indeed I did my doctorate in the early diagnosis of behavioural variant frontotemporal dementia at Cambridge (e.g. Rahman *et al.* 1999). I've also written four books on dementia, so I feel that I am reasonably up to date on the current literature base of dementia and caring globally. That is not to say I would boast that I am an 'expert' in dementia. Indeed, I did not even realise I was a carer to my own mum. I've always considered myself to be primarily the son of my mother, rather than assume any other role.

There are crucial differences you should know about my story at the 'outset'. I am a British Bangladeshi, born in Glasgow, and Mum was born in Bangladesh a long time ago. Ethnic minority groups make up over 14 per cent of the total UK population, many of whom are South Asian (Pakistan, India and Bangladesh), and it is generally acknowledged that there exist difficulties in identifying, diagnosing, and treating dementia in UK ethnic minority groups, including the South Asian population. This is sometimes attributed to low levels of literacy, language barriers and a lack of appropriately translated and culturally adapted screening and diagnostic tools for this ethnic group (Blakemore *et al.* 2018).

The thing is, I don't view my mum most of the time as a person 'living with dementia', either. This is because I am aware of what she has achieved over her lifetime. She came from Bangladesh in the 1960s with her husband, my father, to the UK. She studied education at postgraduate level at Glasgow University, and she has been an amazing, wonderful mother to me. She was always the confident one. She was always the one 'in control'. She always gave me great advice.

There's another reason why I have difficulty in conceptualising her as 'living with dementia'. She is basically the same person to me on the day after she received her diagnosis from the local memory service as she was on the day before. Also, she lives with a number of other conditions, as is common for people living with dementia. The old adage says 'dementia does not travel alone', meaning that dementia is normally accompanied by a number of co-morbidities. She's given me consent to tell you about my lived experience as a carer, and she has been assessed as having mental capacity.

Certain things came to my attention as a result of being her son, as she got to grips with her condition. These were not easy to 'read about' in a textbook, as they were my personal experiences and hers. I should like to explain what I noticed, and throw out for discussion some of the issues. And she doesn't want a 'dementia-friendly community', she tells me, nor to promote one.

The importance of experiences

Inouye (2018) comments:

Who but we can bring value, recognition, and appreciation of older people? We recognize their unique contributions, including wisdom, experience, patience, and resilience. They have lived with adversity and survived with grace and aplomb. They have so much to teach us.

My mum was officially given a diagnosis of dementia about two years ago. Actually, although I did not instigate the line of enquiry, the actual diagnosis came as a relief to me. How did clinicians think she had dementia in the first place? She has consistently performed badly on the Abbreviated Mental Test. She always has been one to change the subject, and talk around stuff. While she came to England in the 1960s, and she feels that her English is very good, I feel that she clearly gets nervous when 'assessed' in formal English. Her first language is Bangladeshi, although she can speak good English. As the dementia has progressed, she prefers to speak in Bangladeshi.

I took my mum on several occasions to hospital, having rung 999. There's an ongoing debate as to whether this was the best thing to do given her frailty and dementia (for example, Voss *et al.* 2018). The presentation makes sense to me looking back on it now. Mum used to take her own medicines. Remember that, until relatively recently, I did not realise Mum lived with dementia – and nor did she. After a meal, where she was sitting down, she would just collapse and fall on the floor. I recollect thinking, while I dialled 999, several times, 'This is it. She's now dying.' Of course, my life would flash in front of my eyes, as I thought, 'This is a moment I'll never forget.' And the 999 call operator would say, 'Try to stay calm. Is she breathing?' After about half a minute, she would thankfully come round and have no recollection of the event. I think looking back on it, Mum had miscounted the volume of anti-hypertensive medications she was meant to take. Of course, the paramedics would do an electrocardiogram (ECG) and check her glucose, and many other essential things – but the journey to the emergency department would normally be quick. That was until one particular admission when she developed a chest infection, and was clearly confused. The consultant geriatrician spotted that she appeared delirious, and as she had fallen on the floor the consultant had requested the CT scan. So, her diagnosis of 'query dementia' essentially came as a result of the acute confusion.

Anyway, the memory clinic prescribed a cholinesterase inhibitor, donepezil. The dementia nurse would speak to me and my mum together. By this time, I had organised with my GP a blister pack so there was no mis-counting of medicines. It was also a useful time to think about pills she really needed, to make it easy for us all.

Being a son caring for my mum encourages me to be 'person-centred', although I have subsequently discovered that paid carers with very little time are somewhat obligated to be task-focused. Having reviewed the literature on this, I find 'person-centred' an overused and rather tired phrase, but I totally get its intentions. But last year, when Mum was admitted with a full-blown delirium, I was truly alerted to how clinicians in hospitals can treat patients without an appreciation of the person attending as a patient. Delirium care for people with dementia to all intents and purposes had become an outpost of veterinary medicine. For example, above the hospital bed, there was a brief summary of the interests of the patient. Above my mum's bed, this list specified 'word searches' and 'listening to music'. I probably visited every day for a few weeks, and puzzled at this list. I used to wonder where 'they' got this information about my mum. The penny dropped when the lead therapist said to my mum one day, 'Would you like to do a word search?' The problem is that the laminated sheet had not been replaced when the last patient had been discharged.

If the basic culture isn't there, it's hard to 'fake it 'til you make it'. Some carers in the previous literature have held the view that hospital care is too task-focused and medically oriented, not delivering treatment in a way that takes individual needs and preferences into account (Douglas-Dunbar and Gardiner 2007). If 'reality orientation' is a means of orienting people with cognitive problems to the world around them, this out-of-date sheet could best be described as 'fiction disorientation'. I suppose that this is what happens when care gets process-managed and happens fast – 'lean' using a best euphemism – but it means that when 'mistakes' occur the emotional feelings which happen can be unnecessarily severe. As a carer, I never wanted to see person-centred care to be so 'tick-boxy', but I suppose that is what will happen when NHS services are under-staffed, under-resourced and working at extremely high pressure.

Learning to accept the diagnosis

As I explained earlier, I never saw myself as a carer.

I have never had any formal training in caring as a carer, and it felt that when I was doing it on my own, I had been plunged in at the deep end. No one told me what I should be doing. No one ever really gave me any feedback on whether my caring was of an acceptable 'standard'. I live with my mum. Therefore, I feel as if I know her really well – possibly better than any other living person. I can therefore tell when 'Mum is not Mum'. I can tell what's unusual for her. I have an instinct for what Mum needs.

I say that guardedly as I had overlooked changes in my mum's ability over the years, and this was in the name of respecting her privacy, autonomy and independence. These were little things. She would get easily lost. She would repeat phrases more often. She lost much of her appetite. I feel embarrassed, looking back on it now, how she wouldn't wish to 'eat her vegetables' or eat the full portion of meat I cooked her a few years back for Christmas dinner. But Mum's ability to look after herself well is a 'biggie'.

Dementia is not as clear-cut as I had been led to believe from my academic training. I passed my diploma of the membership of the Royal Colleges of Physicians in 2005, and my PhD, in dementia, was awarded by Cambridge in 2001. I did not especially seek the diagnosis of dementia. I certainly should have been aware of it given that there has been so much national attention to raising 'dementia awareness' through Dementia Friends, an initiative from the Alzheimer's Society and Public Health England. I even started writing books on dementia in 2014. My first book, *Living Well With Dementia: The Importance of the Person and the Environment*, was even published when I could and should have realised that my mum was developing dementia.

I suppose that events in my life had led me to be in so much denial about her diagnosis. But it was obvious looking back on it. Our GP mentioned to me that he noticed Mum having great difficulty in navigating when coming back from the surgery toilet. I was no longer in denial when Mum failed gloriously in front of me the 'clock drawing test', a bedside test when a person with dementia is requested to draw a clock face and fill the numbers in.

Learning to be a carer

I see myself as a 'care partner', with my mum being 'equal and reciprocal' rather than providing care for my mum on a transactional basis. I still think it's possible to 'care for' someone in the same way you *love* them.

There are little things that make a big difference to me and her. For example, I recently bought her her own mug and saucer, and she handwrote her name on the box, to stamp her territory on it. Of course, investing so much love will one day mean that I feel very hurt at her loss. But we all have to die sometime, and I am determined to celebrate her living. Grief, after all, is a positive emotion if you frame it as the loss of someone you deeply love. If you live with someone '24/7', you learn a lot about the person. But you are not that person. This means that your rights as a carer are not the same as their rights, but complementary.

My conceptualisation of my caring relationship with my mum is much aided by the Carers Trust's Triangle of Care, a working collaboration, or 'therapeutic alliance' between the service user, professional and carer that promotes safety, supports recovery and sustains wellbeing.[1]

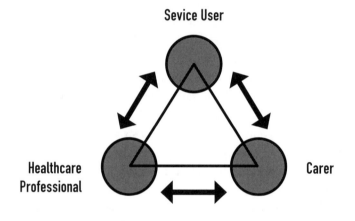

Figure 10.1 Triangle of Care (reproduced by kind permission of the Carers Trust)

Interestingly, 'The Triangle of Care approach was initially developed by carers and staff seeking to improve carer engagement in acute inpatient services' (Carers Trust 2013, p.5).

When somebody you care for is suddenly and unexpectedly admitted to hospital, it can be very disempowering for a person with dementia and their carer. All of the times when Mum has been admitted to a local teaching hospital, there has been no communication with primary care about her direction of travel on care (i.e. the treatment escalation plan). This is nothing new. In clinical situations, the 'shared decision-making model' proposes that clinicians and patients collaborate to make joint decisions based on the best evidence on benefits and harms of all available health options, and on patient values and preferences in regard to those options (Charles, Gafni and Whelan 1999).

I saw this at its worst during Mum's last major admission to hospital. Her cognition and behaviour dropped off a cliff, subsequently referred to,

---

1   www.cwp.nhs.uk/about-us/our-campaigns/person-centred-framework/triangle-of-care

erroneously, by some at the hospital as an 'acute deterioration of dementia'. In fact, the diagnosis was delirium, but, for all the fanciful work around the world about the cognitive assessment of delirium, nobody sought to ask a history from me, the primary carer, about the change I had noticed in my mum. Such poor communication in that hospital had been more than familiar to me when another geriatrician, on a different occasion, looking after my mum said to me on the penultimate day of discharge, 'Oh I didn't realise that you lived with your mother.' Did they really expect that she was living on her own?

A 'delirium-friendly hospital admission'?

A hospital admission of a person with dementia can have a significant impact on the family carer, who temporarily relinquishes caring to health professionals. Using a descriptive qualitative design, holding in-depth interviews with a conversational approach to elicit data, Bloomer *et al.* (2016) found that adjusting to the change in the carer's role can be challenging and result in feelings of helplessness, loneliness, loss of control and being undervalued. Furthermore, there is undeniably a relative scarcity of studies exploring the experience of delirium for patients, carers and families; nevertheless, the studies that do exist raise intriguing questions and possibilities for new therapeutic approaches to improving delirium care for the individual patient (O'Malley *et al.* 2008). While there has been much interest in 'dementia-friendly' environments, in comparison, alarmingly, such environments have received scant attention. When hospitalised, older people, especially with an underlying dementia, can become acutely confused and disorientated. This condition, known as delirium, affects a quarter of older patients.

Delirium is heterogeneous and different aetiologies may have different prognostic implications (Cirbus *et al.* 2018). Delirium in the presence of the pathological processes of dementia is associated with accelerated cognitive decline beyond that expected for delirium or the pathologic process itself. These findings suggest that additional unmeasured pathological processes specifically relate to delirium. Episodes of delirium in people who are not known to have dementia might also reveal dementia at its earliest stages (Davis *et al.* 2017). While both delirium and dementia are important factors in cognitive decline among the elderly, delirium is preventable and treatable through dedicated geriatric care. Further research is needed to understand exactly how delirium interacts with dementia, and how this could be blocked.

Delirium is under-recognised by nurses and is sometimes mistaken for dementia, although delirium can occur in people with dementia, and I feel that appreciating the 'lived experience' of people who've had delirum, and their carers, is critical.

There are broadly three types of delirium:[2]

- *Hyperactive delirium:* Probably the most easily recognised type, this may include restlessness (e.g. pacing), agitation, rapid mood changes or hallucinations, and refusal to cooperate with care.
- *Hypoactive delirium:* This may include inactivity or reduced motor activity, sluggishness, abnormal drowsiness, or seeming to be in a daze.
- *Mixed delirium:* This includes both hyperactive and hypoactive signs and symptoms. The person may quickly switch back and forth from hyperactive to hypoactive states.

In addition, 'subsyndromal delirium' is thought to represent a sub-threshold state related to delirium and associated with poor post-hospitalisation outcomes similar to those associated with delirium (Levkoff *et al.*1996).

Mum had a protracted hospital admission due to delirium at the beginning of 2018. It was characterised by hypoactive delirium, which was really scary to me as I did not know what it was nor how long it would last. I now realise that we actually know very little about the neuroscience of delirium, full stop. I found the whole experience very distressing, especially since I was told nothing about how or when mum would get better, what was causing her symptoms, and what to expect. That was all compounded by a 'shotgun' notice to think about transferring Mum to a residential setting on discharge.

Delirium is still associated with high rates of institutionalisation and an increased risk of death up to five years after the index event; prior to delirium, individuals seem to compensate for their vulnerability (Eeles *et al.* 2010). Moving a relative or friend with dementia into a care home can be a difficult decision to make for anyone, and it can be emotional for both the person with dementia and their family and friends.[3] Making the decision in an emergency situation is not a particularly good idea either, especially when you don't know what the future brings. As it happened, Mum came home with me, and we continue to live together. She and I could not be

---

2   www.mayoclinic.org/diseases-conditions/delirium/symptoms-causes/syc-20371386

3   www.dementiauk.org/preparing-move-care-home

happier – though it is hard work. I would defend the 'Home First'[4] initiative, therefore, to the hilt.

I felt at the time that my experience of Mum with delirium in hospital was bad, but it was only when I started reading around the area that I discovered how bad it was. The Royal College of Physicians' (2006) guidelines on delirium were intended 'to provide hospital doctors, nurses, allied health professionals, care assistants, commissioners of services, relatives and carers with a practical approach to the identification, prevention and management of delirium'.[5] While the guidelines were apparently developed primarily with a view to hospital care, the principles within the guidelines are also highly relevant to intermediate and community care settings. I do, however, sympathise with clinical staff, who can easily find themselves in totally unfamiliar territory. Nurses are, arguably, the staff in most frequent and intimate contact with patients, and it is generally acknowledged that caring for delirious patients may be difficult, stressful and, at times, dangerous (Hallberg 1999). And I certainly don't envy their uphill task with this admission. Although I felt somewhat like a 'secret shopper', Mum's admission to this 'world class' hospital was educational. Overriding everything else, a perceived lack of dignity and respect towards patients with dementia has been a genuine concern for me.

Let me consider some of the points in those guidelines.

1. Keep the use of sedatives and major tranquillisers to a minimum.
2. One-to-one care of the patient is often required.
3. Restraints (including cotsides, 'geriatric chairs', etc.) have not been shown to prevent falls and may increase the risk of injury. It may be preferable to nurse the patient on a low bed or place the mattress directly on the floor. Adoption of the good practices described should make the use of physical restraints unnecessary for the management of confusion.
4. Assessment by a physiotherapist and occupational therapist to maintain and improve functional ability should be considered in all delirious patients.
5. A full continence assessment should be carried out. Regular toileting and prompt treatment of urinary tract infections may prevent urinary incontinence. Catheters should be avoided where possible

---

4 https://fabnhsstuff.net/fab-stuff/developing-home-first-mindset-liz-sargeant

5 www.rcplondon.ac.uk/guidelines-policy/
   prevention-diagnosis-referral-and-management-delirium-older-people

because of the increased risks of trauma in confused patients, and the risk of catheter-associated infection.

6. Senior doctors and nurses should ensure that doctors in training and nurses are able to recognise and treat delirium.

Royal College of Physicians' guidelines on delirium – some selected points for discussion

The neuropsychopharmacology of delirium is poorly understood. I would find that, with no explanation, a nurse would administer an injection intramuscularly, while Mum was sleeping. When I then enquired what the injection was, after a bit of time I found out it was lorazepam, a benzodiazepine. It has long been appreciated that drugs have been associated with the development of delirium in the elderly. Successful treatment of delirium depends on identifying the reversible contributing factors, and drugs are the most common reversible cause of delirium.

Polypharmacy in people living with dementia has been linked to higher risks of hospitalisation and death in community samples. It is commonly present in people with dementia but these risks have rarely been studied in this population (Mueller *et al.* 2018). Anticholinergic medications, benzodiazepines and narcotics in high doses are common causes of drug-induced delirium (Alagiakrishnan and Wiens 2004). As a result of deprescribing all my mum's medications, the cholinesterase inhibitor, donepezil, was suddenly withdrawn, and I have absolutely no doubt that this made her delirium considerably worse. Also, it was incredibly distressing for me, as everyone in the bay had medications in the nurse-led drug round, except my mum. With no explanation as to how this had happened, even though I had made myself available on the consultant ward round, I assumed that the medical team were now withdrawing all medication in some end-of-life bid. This is just one of countless examples where there was ridiculously bad communication with the carer. Simply sticking a John's Campaign[6] poster up on the wall is not really good enough.

Mum was already sleeping due to hypoactive delirium, so this made the delirium worse. Regardless of your legal opinions on paternalism and the doctrine of necessity, there's an argument that this physical assault was not in my mum's best interests. Talking of which, no clinical staff bothered to clarify with me that I was the lasting power of attorney for health and welfare,

---

6   John's Campaign is a campaign for extended visiting rights for family carers of patients with dementia in hospitals in the UK, founded in November 2014

something which took me aeons to organise as I was given very little help from both primary and secondary care. So, I discovered that, whatever you are told at these dementia conferences, this is the *actual reality* of 'dementia rights'. Maybe as a result of paternalism, there was no 'shared decision making', and Mum and I felt that we had no rights in this hospital admission for delirium.

Mum had a bedrail on this admission – even though she was sleeping all the time. Why? I feel that Oliver (2002) was extremely insightful to bring this issue up ahead of his time:

> The European Human Rights Act 2000 may in time add to the complexity of such cases – as there is a provision that 'no-one shall be subjected to inhuman or degrading treatment' – which might potentially be interpreted either way in the application or non-application of bedrails. What we can say is that whilst there is a duty of care on the hospital to provide a safe environment, there is not a duty to protect from all conceivable risks and that restraint against the will of a mentally competent patient could constitute an assault or civil wrong. (Oliver 2002)

There was no one-to-one care, and, when I have seen it done for other patients in other hospitals, this 'specialing' has made it appear as if the person with dementia is a serious criminal offender. This does make me feel extremely uneasy about the way society, and services in general, 'treat' people and patients with dementia. Even though Mum was sleeping all the time, and showed no interest in eating or drinking, there was no one-to-one care, apart from at mealtimes, when thankfully a healthcare assistant would try to help. But they were invariably somehow doing one-to-one feeding with more than one patient at once, and there was a very low threshold for judging that the 'patient refused' when no one had helped mum to take the polythene wrapping off the microwaved hospital meal. Mum with delirium, having been going to the toilet before, was immediately put into incontinence pads, because there was no motivation to answer her buzzer or 'mobilise her' to the toilet. A frequent complaint in the literature has been a failure of the hospital to provide for basic personal care needs, including help with washing, dressing, toileting, eating, drinking or taking medication. Omissions in basic care provision are partly attributed to a lack of understanding and compassion on the part of the staff, although low staffing levels are also cited (Beardon *et al.* 2018). For the record, mum has been in incontinence pads ever since – what I call 'iatrogenic incontinence'. I was saddened when culturally it was deemed much easier to keep mum bedbound for the whole of her admission across weeks, apart from one or two tokenistic efforts to sit her by the window.

Disuse of the muscles leads to atrophy and a loss of muscle strength at a rate of around 12 per cent a week (Jiricka 2008). After three to five weeks of bedrest, almost half the normal strength of a muscle is lost. 'End PJ Paralysis' was non-existent (for an explanation of #EndPJParalyis, see this blogpost[7]), which meant that she not only lost muscle bulk, but we both lost confidence, and she unsurprisingly was discharged with a hoist (which she has never used to this day). Watching your mum lying in bed all day, while she is ignored by the therapists, is distressing for the carer. Of course, to be fair, the therapists will wish to argue that Mum was unable to comply with requests for therapy as she was so delirious.

It would have been pointless asking any of the medical staff about delirium. The consultant geriatrician could barely answer my questions, and I don't think the junior doctors even recognised the delirium. No clinician mentioned the word 'delirium' on ward rounds, until I brought it up. It did not even appear on the final discharge summary. So, Mum was eventually discharged, not eating or drinking properly, and not walking either. Luckily, with her return to a home environment, her delirium 'lifted', and she slowly returned to some normality via what I think was a 'subsyndromal delirium'. Subsyndromal delirium is a clinical term usually defined as the presence of one or more symptoms of delirium, not meeting criteria for delirium and not progressing to delirium. This means the patient has some but not all of the symptoms of delirium and may be quite significantly affected but still not clinically have delirium. I have subsequently found out from one of my Twitter followers, Professor Sharon Inouye at Harvard University, that recovery through a subsyndromal phase is quite common (through her unpublished data.)

Conclusion

I am indeed proud of all professionals, including clinicians, but I do feel, reluctantly, that the overall culture does not value carers. I also never fail to be amazed by the 'silo mentality' within health and social care sectors – especially concerning a cultural inability to embrace the idea that professionals can

---

7   www.england.nhs.uk/2018/03/70-days-to-end-pyjama-paralysis

be informal carers too. I've long felt that anything can happen to anyone at any time, but I personally wouldn't wish dementia on anyone. I dare say it is possible to 'live well with dementia', but really it is time to stop airbrushing out people with advanced dementia from important 'engagement'. Commissioning practices need to swing this pendulum away. It was telling for me that 'caring well' did not feature in conference talks on dementia, whereas other themes such as 'supporting well' and 'diagnosing well' *were* represented. I've really resented what dementia has done to my mum, but I fundamentally feel that she is still the person I've always known. I owe my life to her, quite literally, and it is my duty, especially given my clinical, research and legal training, to look after her in her time of need now. That duty, however, is above all as her son.

Acknowledgement

I would like to thank my mum who gave her full informed consent for this chapter to be published.

References

Alagiakrishnan, K. and Wiens, C.A. (2004) 'An approach to drug induced delirium in the elderly.' *Postgraduate Medical Journal*, 80, 945, 388–393.

Beardon, S., Patel, K., Davies, B. and Ward, H. (2018) 'Informal carers' perspectives on the delivery of acute hospital care for patients with dementia: A systematic review.' *BMC Geriatrics*, 18, 1, 23. doi: 10.1186/s12877-018-0710-x.

Blakemore, A., Kenning, C., Mirza, N., Daker-White, G., Panagioti, M. and Waheed, W. (2018) 'Dementia in UK South Asians: A scoping review of the literature.' *BMJ Open*, 8, 4: e020290. doi: 10.1136/bmjopen-2017-020290.

Bloomer, M., Digby, R., Tan, H., Crawford, K. and Williams, A. (2016) 'The experience of family carers of people with dementia who are hospitalised.' *Dementia (London)*, 15, 5, 1234–1245. doi: 10.1177/1471301214558308. Epub 13 November 2014.

Carers Trust (2013) *The Triangle of Care. Carers Included: A Guide to Best Practice in Mental Health Care in England* (second edition). London: Carers Trust. Available at: https://professionals.carers.org/sites/default/files/thetriangleofcare_guidetobestpracticeinmentalhealthcare_england.pdf.

Charles, C., Gafni, A. and Whelan, T. (1999) 'Decision-making in the physician-patient encounter: revisiting the shared treatment decision-making model.' *Social Science & Medicine*, 49, 5, 651–661.

Cirbus, J., MacLullich, A., Noel, C., Ely, E., Chandrasekhar, R. and Han, J. (2018) 'Delirium etiology subtypes and their effect on six-month function and cognition in older emergency department patients.' *International Psychogeriatrics*, 1–10. doi:10.1017/S1041610218000777.

Davis, D.H., Muniz-Terrera, G., Keage, H.A., Stephan, B.C. *et al.* (2017) 'Epidemiological Clinicopathological Studies in Europe (EClipSE) Collaborative Members. Association of delirium with cognitive decline in late life: A neuropathologic study of 3 population-based cohort studies.' *JAMA Psychiatry*, 74, 3, 244–251. doi: 10.1001/jamapsychiatry.2016.3423.

Douglas-Dunbar, M. and Gardiner, P. (2007) 'Support for carers of people with dementia during hospital admission.' *Nursing Older People*, 19, 8, 27–30.

Eeles, E.M., Hubbard, R.E., White, S.V., O'Mahony, M.S., Savva, G.M. and Bayer, A.J. (2010) 'Hospital use, institutionalisation and mortality associated with delirium.' *Age and Ageing*, 39, 4, 470–475. doi: 10.1093/ageing/afq052.

Hallberg, I.R. (1999) 'Impact of delirium on professionals.' *Dementia and Geriatric Cognitive Disorders*, 10, 420–425.

Inouye, S.K. (2018) 'Delirium: A framework to improve acute care for older persons.' *Journal of the American Geriatrics Society*, 66, 3, 446–451. doi: 10.1111/jgs.15296. Epub 23 February 2018.

Jiricka, M.K. (2008) 'Activity Tolerance and Fatigue Pathophysiology: Concepts of Altered Health States.' In C.M. Porth (ed.) *Essentials of Pathophysiology: Concepts of Altered Health States*. Philadelphia, PA: Lippincott Williams & Wilkins.

Levkoff, S.E., Liptzin, B., Cleary, P.D., Wetle, T., Evans, D.A. and Rowe, J.W. (1996) 'Subsyndromal delirium.' *American Journal of Geriatric Psychiatry*, 4, 320–329.

Mueller, C., Molokhia, M., Perera, G., Veronese, N. *et al.* (2018) 'Polypharmacy in people with dementia: Associations with adverse health outcomes.' *Experimental Gerontology*, 106, 240–245. doi: 10.1016/j.exger.2018.02.011. Epub 13 February 2018.

Oliver, D. (2002) 'Hobby Horse. Bed falls and bedrails – what should we do?' *Age and Ageing*, 31, 415–418.

O'Malley, G., Leonard, M., Meagher, D. and O'Keeffe, S.T. (2008) 'The delirium experience: a review.' *Journal of Psychosomatic Research*, 65, 3, 223–228. doi: 10.1016/j.jpsychores.2008.05.017.

Rahman, S., Sahakian, B.J., Hodges, J.R., Rogers, R.D. and Robbins, T.W. (1999) 'Specific cognitive deficits in mild frontal variant frontotemporal dementia.' *Brain*, 122 (Pt 8), 1469–1493.

Royal College of Physicians (2006) *Concise Guidance to Good Practice: A Series of Evidence-Based Guidelines for Clinical Management. Number 6: The Prevention, Diagnosis and Management of Delirium in Older People. National Guidelines*. London: Royal College of Physicians.

Voss, S., Brandling, J., Taylor, H., Black, S. *et al.* (2018) 'How do people with dementia use the ambulance service? A retrospective study in England: The HOMEWARD project.' *BMJ Open*, 1, 8, 7, e022549. doi: 10.1136/bmjopen-2018-022549.

CHAPTER 11

Summary

David Truswell

The preceding chapters have looked as some key commonalities in the impact of dementia across Black, Asian and minority ethnic communities (BAME) and explored in some detail both current academic research and the experience of dementia within a number of communities through testimony from experience from those living with dementia or those caring for people living with dementia. Authors such as Banarjee (2015) have argued for some time that dementia is inherently a complex phenomenon usually involving multiple physical co-morbidities. Family carers of people living with dementia often point out that supporting someone living with dementia is more challenging than other forms of caring as the personality changes and increasing cognitive impairment impact on the relationship with the carer and others in a way some have described as a 'bereavement' while the person felt to have been lost is physically still alive. Cultural background adds a further level of complexity to the psychological and social impact of dementia for the person living with dementia, and their family and social network, and this has an impact at all stages of living with dementia.

An individual's ideas about their cultural identity sit at the centre of their sense of themselves and are important anchoring points for memory and identity as other reference points become harder to keep hold of. These reference points of cultural identity are likely to be highly personalised, and in providing personalised dementia care, understanding the person must involve more than approaching care and support of people from a BAME background armed with a rigid cultural checklist. The character of first-generation migrants will have been forged through early childhood experience outside the UK and they are likely to have found their lifetime experience in the UK has often seen their cultural identity contested or treated as adversarial, intrusive or marginalised. It should be expected that when living with dementia their personal ideas about cultural identity may be some of the most emotionally strong and psychologically resonant points of connection and communication. As families move through second, third and later migrant generations, the individual significance of cultural identity and the form it takes will change.

The challenge for personalising the care of people living with dementia from BAME communities is understanding the cultural and personal significance of events, objects, music and other materials through their eyes, a significance that may not be fully appreciated even by family carers. There may be life events and psychologically resonant incidents that they have never spoken of to their children. Their story of themselves in their culture in the UK is not the same as their children's. Regardless of the circumstances of migration, the decision to migrate is a major psychological step that takes the migrant beyond their previous cultural circumstances. The psychological displacement and experience of alienation and discrimination that are part of the cultural experience of migration are rarely referenced in the general appeal for more 'cultural competence' by dementia services.

There are increased risks of dementia for the African-Caribbean and South Asian populations that need to be better understood and may be modifiable through preventative measures. There is sufficient evidence for a sustained dementia-awareness campaign targeting these communities; continued institutional complacency about the under-representation in services and increased risk for these populations needs to be more forcefully challenged. The broader picture of lifetime risk of poor health for the Irish and Gypsy and Traveller communities argues for more research on the impact of dementia on these communities. The current information gap is startling given the size and age demographic of the Irish community in the UK.

Far more recognition needs to be given to locality-based work being done by community groups that clearly secures the emotional investment and support of communities and should be sustained and built on far more fruitfully than endless rounds of consultation with BAME groups, which result in sustained inaction. Examples in this book from the Chinese National Healthy Living Association and Jewish Care illustrate comprehensive approaches to support organised at a scale to deliver effective outcomes that people in the respective communities value. Often the learning from this kind of work, including developing materials that are appropriate to the respective communities, is lost due to short-term funding and a lack of infrastructure to collate and disseminate any information, reports or materials generated.

One does not see much reporting of localities using the NHS *Plan, Do, Study Act* (ACT Academy 2018) model of service development to follow through from small pilots looking at dementia and BAME communities, and scale up and sustain the learning from the pilot either into larger numbers within the community involved in the pilot or larger numbers across communities that may respond to similar interventions. Initiatives such as Community Action on Dementia in Brent[1] do seem to be taking this approach and working closely with local commissioners in their development. However, elsewhere initiatives such as that of Liverpool Dementia Action Alliance,[2] which seemed to be making impressive strides in developing a multi-community approach to dementia, including developing dementia awareness video materials for a variety of communities and community dementia champions, are being defunded. This is more typical of the fate of BAME community developments currently. Similar threats of funding loss are faced by Touchstone in Leeds and Meri Yaadain, despite having been developing their work for some years and having received national-level recognition.

There is little evidence that the expertise of community organisations or the voice of lived experience from people from BAME communities living with dementia, and their family carers, is particularly successfully sought out by the dementia mainstream, despite the demographic risk issues for some communities identified earlier in this book. The increasing representation of images of people of colour at almost every level of contemporary dementia documentation for the general public contrasts with the paucity of contribution in those same documents from the diverse voices of people from BAME backgrounds and the lack of appropriate service provision identified for BAME communities. This is more disconcerting as we know there will be a seven-fold increase in the number of people from BAME communities based on age profile alone (All Party Parliamentary Group on Dementia 2013). It is likely to be even greater when the factor of increased risk for some communities is considered.

Dementia may be experienced as not only a profound illness but also as a challenge to faith and spirituality by the person living with dementia and/or by those close to them and caring for them in a way that other illnesses may not be similarly experienced. As faith and spirituality play such an important part in the lives of many from BAME communities, it is prudent that service providers should be mindful that this can often be a significant issue for

---

1   www.cad-brent.org.uk

2   www.youtube.com/channel/UCIdiZ9ZXxcsqbF9ES-96w5Q

someone living with dementia, and their partners and family. This does not require service personnel simply to have a ready checklist of all religions at the point of first contact but to understand the need to have a conversation about faith and belief and people's wishes and preferences related to this in the context of planning their care and support.

From the human rights and dementia perspective, the important development of dementia rights in the UK needs to have a nuanced agenda that responds to BAME communities as a vulnerable group needing particular focus on being informed of their rights and enabled to exercise them. In the UK's political climate that contests the health service access of migrants, BAME people with dementia will be potentially faced with additional problems in not simply accessing healthcare but insisting on their access to equitable health and care, as will their family carers and advocates who attempt to insist on this access on their behalf. United Nations Human Rights Commission guidelines (International Organization for Migration 2007) are quite clear in identifying the rights of vulnerable groups as a priority requiring focused support in the implementation of human rights initiatives and identify ethnic minorities as one of the vulnerable groups. It is not evident that the current approach to dementia and human rights in the UK fully takes this on board as an issue of priority underpinned by vulnerability rather than simply an additional extra issue on the UK dementia rights agenda. This is an issue that needs much stronger advocacy within the dementia rights perspective in the UK and one hopes that the analysis in this book by Toby Williamson and other contributions elsewhere such as that of Truswell (2018) help to emphasise this.

Interpreting is often more complex in dementia settings than interpreting in other medical settings, and building trust between the person living with dementia, family members, professional interpreter and the dementia professional is essential. It is the responsibility of the clinical professional to take the lead in this. However, creating this trusting working relationship and developing the broader skillset required to work confidently with interpreters is something dementia professionals and care staff should have training in rather than simply be expected to acquire on the job through trial and error.

There are shortcomings in the standard diagnostic assessment tools that may distort the degree of assessed cognitive impairment, but progress to date in identifying and evaluating more reliable cross-culturally validated assessment tools is limited (Wood *et al.* 2006) and there is no nationally agreed recommended diagnostic tool that overcomes these shortcomings.

Reminiscence material appropriate for the history of people from BAME backgrounds is in short supply. The lack of culturally appropriate provision in dementia not only has implications for the quality of care but also creates additional costs for people from BAME communities for routine aspects of care and support in mainstream services, such as personal hygiene and nutrition, when BAME families must directly finance these costs for routine aspects of care.

The dictum of that 'once you have met one person with dementia, you have met one person with dementia' holds for BAME communities too, in both the case of the person living with dementia, and those who may be their main carer(s). Cultural expectations change over time and the act of migration itself has an impact on the migrants' understanding of themselves in relation to their culture. Many long-standing BAME communities in the UK that are not mentioned in this book have similar issues with dementia and access to services. These may be communities such as the Polish with a large national presence across the UK, but also smaller migrant communities such as the Vietnamese, Cypriot, Tamil, Italian, Afghani, Somali, Spanish and Orthodox Jewish, to name just a few. These may be locally numerous or dispersed, reflecting the communities' migration history and the historic development of UK migration policy. As future migrant communities settle and grow old in the UK, it is important to build and sustain the skillset of staff and continuity of practice development. This will enable staff to respond to and understand the cultural complexities this can introduce into dementia care as a routine element of thinking about the planning of care, rather than treating each newly ageing community as a novel emergence at the margins that creates 'cultural' problems for services.

Dementia is the most significant global challenge to the world's healthcare economy thus far in the 21st century. It is a complex and terminal illness with profound psychological implications not just for those living with dementia but for all those close to them. The psychological, economic and physical challenges that family members, loved ones and close friends caring for people living with dementia face are little researched. The complexities carers deal with as a result of people living with dementia, who often have other physical problems that need ongoing treatment, are often not appreciated; thus carers themselves are untrained and unsupported in managing the often complex care needs they encounter. They also do not have the professional psychological and social support infrastructure available to dementia professionals and paid care staff. The psychological and health risk issues linked to stress, overwork and the lack of timely breaks from the work of caring, which in employment are covered by the employers 'duty of care', are less examined in the case of carers. There are studies that suggest that BAME carers from some communities may experience more carer burden compared with White UK carers (Parveen and Oyebode 2018) but the research picture is mixed as there are so few studies.

Mainstream media portrayals of dementia routinely involve characters who are living with no health problems other than dementia, and often show dementia that involves little in the way of bewildering personality changes, mood changes or aggressive or disinhibited behaviour of the kind mentioned by a number of contributors to this book. For BAME carers and those living with dementia from BAME backgrounds, their cultural values and beliefs add further complexity to living with dementia as they struggle to understand what is happening, seek help and diagnosis and try to put in place appropriate supporting care and services through to the end of life.

While there are some broad general features that have been identified in this book that are likely to affect the experience of living with dementia across all BAME communities, there are also some specific features for some communities that can be materially important for understanding and managing the experience of living with dementia for people from those communities. However, at the individual level, every person or family's experience of living with dementia is unique. People will vary in the way they feel about their cultural/family obligations and expectations and in their practical ability to act on how they feel in their own personal circumstances. Room for negotiation of who will care and what this will involve will vary highly within the dynamics of families. Within culturally mixed relationships, families may be quite fluid in their understanding of culturally held expectations of care for elders.

Cultural matching may bring important cultural knowledge into the care provision for those living with dementia, but it can also bring unhelpful cultural preconceptions about dementia too. Contributions from personal experience in this book identify strong and positive bonds built up between paid carers and people living with dementia from different ethnic backgrounds. Jewish Care, for example, does well-respected and culturally validating work within the Jewish community, employing many staff who are not Jewish as there is an excellent programme of education in understanding Jewish religion and culture for staff. Authors and educators such as Dr Karan Jutlla have for some time pointed out the fallacy of assuming that the South Asian community is homogenous and that cultural matching is synonymous with providing good care which is culturally appropriate for the person living with dementia.

Pulling together perspectives and material presented in this book, a number of key actions are proposed that would help to secure a much-needed improvement in dementia service information, access and support for those in UK BAME communities living with dementia, and their families and carers. These are:

1. A national-level repository of information and resources should be created which brings together the formal research and broader learning and localised work taking place through community organisations. This Resource Hub needs to have a live connection to BAME community organisations to collate reports, materials and good practice examples nationwide. The management and advisory structure of the Resource Hub should include significant representation from BAME community organisations working with dementia. It would not only provide a collection point for developments that might otherwise reside in the so-called 'grey literature' (or increasing only on a YouTube channel) but also act as an advisory resource and dissemination point. The Resource Hub would have a development interface with the NHS to explore how projects that evidence improvements in the experience and outcomes of dementia services by people from BAME communities living with dementia, and their carers, can be scaled up to cover broader populations locally or nationally.

2. A commitment should be made, linked to resource and funding investment, into targeting and prioritising information about dementia to the demographically higher risk BAME groups. Community organisations need to be recruited into supporting the provision of this information through local community outlets as well as making information made available through the mainstream. The anticipated seven-fold increase in the numbers of people from BAME groups living with dementia will proportionally impact more on the demographically older BAME groups.

3. It should be recognised that BAME carers are potentially at risk of becoming socially isolated, through ostracism as a result of stigma or as a result of cultural traditions valuing 'strong mindedness' and independence that lead them to feel they have to care on their own or can only call on help from within the family. Carers are unlikely to understand the complexities and long-term nature of

the support they are undertaking and have little access to support mechanisms for themselves. There needs to be a sea change in the understanding BAME communities have of dementia – one that mobilises inclusion and community resilience in support both of people living with dementia, and their carers. BAME carers are key to the delivery of good care for BAME people living with dementia. There needs to be a focus on how BAME communities are being helped to look after BAME people living with dementia and how BAME carers are supported with this, not continuing the institutional stereotyped and biased view that it happens magically as 'people look after their own'. This needs to be led by and through BAME community organisations and not only incorporate training and support for carers but also enable and develop community resilience and social capital within the communities.

4. A better understanding needs to be developed of the additional personal costs incurred by those from the BAME communities for aspects of care provision that are part of routine care and support. Examples of this might be haircare and other aspects of personal care, diet and nutritional supplements, and access to ministry. As tax payers and citizens, BAME families and BAME community organisations should not be providing an unacknowledged supplement for routine aspects of service provision from dementia services as a result of failures in the provision of equity in health and social care in older people's public services.

5. There should be a requirement that to obtain funding for dementia research, UK research organisations must show how they will actively work to include BAME communities in their dementia work. In the US, federally funded research often requires research organisations to demonstrate how the work they are doing has included participation of diverse communities before they are eligible for programme funds (Sheikh *et al.* 2009). Some similar constraint in funding for dementia research could encourage UK research organisations to actively work to include BAME communities in dementia research. Sheikh *et al.* (2009) identify UK research organisations as institutionally reluctant to engage with BME populations on research. More recently, Truswell (2019) has drawn attention to a number of researchers offering a critique of

the research communities' marginalisation of members of BAME communities as research participants.

6. Hypothecating a modest proportion (10%) of dementia research funding to non-pharmacological interventions in dementia would enormously benefit this research and has far more potential to encourage engagement of BAME research participants. A powerful narrative trope that is highly influential in much of the mainstream media is the pharmacological 'cure for dementia' that scientists are often portrayed as being on the verge of discovering. The problems with this almost religious belief in a pharmacological miracle have been articulated in Truswell (2017) but one feature of this argument for a pharmacological miracle is that people living with dementia now seem to be expected to simply wait for it to arrive, with little else offered in the interim. As pharmacological trials continue to fail (Mullane and Williams 2013), there are a number socially based interventions that at small scale seem to be delivering significant improvements in clinical symptoms and quality of life with modest and non-invasive methodologies. These methodologies have no negative pharmacological side effects. Many of these methodologies involve structured intervention of various kinds – dementia navigators, children in residential units, music, 'Singing for the Brain', dance, physical contact (e.g. pets or robot pet substitutes) or digital imaging – and most lend themselves to cross-cultural implementation (Ronzi *et al.* 2018). These seem to be producing more evidenced clinical and social benefit for people living with dementia than we have recently seen from the pharmacological field. There needs to be a shift in favour of more funding to support research into these approaches.

7. There needs to be much more participation and active challenge in the UK from those in BAME communities regarding the equitable provision of dementia services and support for people from BAME communities living with dementia, and their carers. The past five years since the signature high-level policy investigation document *Dementia does not discriminate* (All Party Parliamentary Group on Dementia 2013) have seen very little development in information and provision in what may be one of the most serious health changes currently facing BAME communities.

At the highest level of UK dementia policy, it should be recognised that policy documents such *Prime Minister's Challenge on Dementia 2020: Implementation Plan* (Dementia Policy Team 2016) and previous high-level policy documents have consistently highlighted the importance of some of the issues for BAME communities and other disadvantaged groups. This has in principle already had a measure of focus at the highest level. However, the delivery of these high-level national strategic intentions regarding BAME communities has floundered more at the regional and local level over the ten years since the first National Dementia Strategy (Department of Health 2009), despite some thoughtful and insightful initiatives led by local leaders with strong personal commitments to this agenda, whether within the research community or local health and care systems. Many of these initiatives have been isolated, local and piecemeal, hardly reflecting the national priority or the national demographic challenge. The continued lack of action nationally and regionally to sustain, consolidate and support leaves these local initiatives isolated in their dependence on committed individuals. This hardly constitutes a reasoned national strategy for the identified raised risk of dementia in these demographically identifiable BAME communities, which may well be amenable to some modification through lifestyle and diet changes. With a little imagination, this could also be integrated with other current health improvement strategies for BAME communities, such as diabetes, smoking cessation and heart disease.

Those people from BAME communities living with dementia who are not known to services or only come to achieve service contact at the later stages of their illness are already living in the community. They are more likely to arrive in services in severe distress with multiple health and social issues – through emergency departments with delirium, infection (urinary or pulmonary) or a fracture as a result of fall – and then are found to be living with dementia, complicating both the treatment of the admitting issue and discharge. They may also arrive in services as complex emergency health and care cases as a result of breakdown of informal care arrangements as carers become 'burnt out', isolated and unable to cope.

These crisis cases absorb far more time and are more costly to resolve than a consistent, proactively managed approach across the system that recognises the importance of cultural elements in the provision of effective and appropriate dementia care. This requires an approach that integrates thinking about cultural aspects of the provision in health information and public education, assessment and diagnosis, support service arrangements and on through to end-of-life care. It also involves enabling strengths in the family and social relationships of the person living with dementia to encourage retaining social inclusion, and working with community organisations to mobilise resilience through community support and understanding. Most dementia care and support takes place in the community (Department of Health 2013) and for many areas of the UK communities there is a local demographic ethnic mix that includes a substantial proportion of BAME elders living with dementia. This proportion will increase.

While there are, and will continue to be, some significant initiatives at local level to improve access and the quality of dementia services for BAME communities, these are often isolated and short-lived. They need to be built on with sustained and adequately funded action within an appropriate, supporting national and regional infrastructure that encourages and builds on local good practice and facilitates rapid dissemination of what has been learned in other areas. It is time to stop reinventing the wheel and get on with building the bicycle so we can all actually get somewhere.

References

ACT Academy (2018) *Plan, Do, Study, Act (PDSA) Cycles and the Model for Improvement.* NHS Improvement. Available at: https://improvement.nhs.uk/documents/2142/plan-do-study-act.pdf [accessed 01/12/2018].

All Party Parliamentary Group on Dementia (2013) *Dementia does not discriminate: The experiences of black, Asian and minority ethnic communities.* London: All Party Parliamentary Group on Dementia.

Banerjee, S. (2015) 'Multimorbidity – older adults need health care that can count past one.' *The Lancet*, 385, 587–589.

Dementia Policy Team (2016) *Prime Minister's Challenge on Dementia 2020: Implementation Plan.* Available at: www.gov.uk/government/publications/challenge-on-dementia-2020-implementation-plan [accessed 28/01/2019].

Department of Health (2009) *Living Well with Dementia: A National Dementia Strategy.* London: Department of Health.

Department of Health (2013) *Dementia: A state of the nation report on dementia care and support in England.* London: Department of Health.

International Organization for Migration (2007) *International Migration, Health and Human Rights.* Le Grand-Saconnex, Switzerland: International Organization for Migration.

Mullane, K. and Williams, M. (2013) 'Alzheimer's therapeutics: Continued clinical failures question the validity of the amyloid hypothesis – but what lies beyond?' *Biochemical Pharmacology*, 85, 289–305.

Parveen, S. and Obeyode, J. (2018) *Dementia and Ethnic Minority Carers' Better Health Briefing, 46.* Race Equality Foundation.

Ronzi, S., Orton, L., Pope, D., Valtorta, N. and Bruce, N. (2018) 'What is the impact on health and wellbeing of interventions that foster respect and social inclusion in community-residing older adults? A systematic review of quantitative and qualitative studies.' *Systematic Reviews, 7*, 26.

Sheikh, A., Halani, L., Bhopal, R., Netuveli, G. *et al.* (2009) 'Facilitating the recruitment of minority ethnic people into research: Qualitative case study of South Asians and asthma.' *PLoS Med, 6*, 10, e1000148. doi:10.1371/journal.pmed.1000148.

Truswell, D. (2017) 'Dementia: faith in science or faith in pharmacy.' *Journal of Dementia, 1*, 1: e101.

Truswell, D. (2018) 'Dementia, Human Rights and BME communities.' *Journal of Dementia Care, 25*, 1, 22–23.

Truswell, D. (2019) *Black, Asian and Minority Ethnic Communities and Dementia – 5 Years On.* London: Race Equality Foundation.

Wood, R.Y., Giuliano, K.K., Bignell, C.U. and Pritham, W.W. (2006) 'Assessing cognitive ability in research: Use of MMSE with minority populations and elderly adults with low education levels.' *Journal of Gerontological Nursing, 32*, 4, 45–54.

BAME and Dementia Resources

Alzheimer's Society
www.alzheimers.org.uk
The Alzheimer's Society has a strong tradition of working with BAME community groups to improve dementia information and services for BAME communities and is a good online information resource for research and reports on dementia in Black and minority ethnic (BME) communities.

BME Health and Wellbeing
www.bmehaw.co.uk
A community group based in Rochdale that supports people from the BME and South Asian communities. It is very active in campaigning and encouraging local BAME populations to become involved in health research.

Chinese National Healthy Living
www.cnhlc.org.uk/zhangs-story
The Chinese National Healthy Living Centre completed a five-year project at the end of 2018 on raising awareness about dementia in the Chinese community in London. The project reached across several London boroughs and culminated in the Centre organising the first UK conference on dementia in the Chinese community to include a live transmission link to a Chinese community group in the North of England. It also provides information on dementia in Chinese.

Culture Dementia UK
www.culturedementiauk.org
An organisations that has been working in Brent for the past 15 years, initially with the African-Caribbean community, but has expanded to cover awareness-raising, advice and support to many communities.

Dementia Alliance for Culture and Ethnicity
www.demace.com
An alliance of groups that provides information and support to people from BAME communities in the UK. The website includes a number of video resources for raising awareness about dementia in BAME communities.

Dementia Diversity Xchange Network (DDXN)
www.ddxn.org.uk
Reflecting the emergence of a grassroots attempt to create a more regional infrastructure to explore the impact of dementia across BAME communities, the creation of this hub organisation in the Midlands supports the development of the BAME and dementia evidence base.

Dementia UK
www.dementiauk.org
A national charity which promotes and develops Admiral Nursing, a specialist nursing intervention focused on meeting the needs of families and people with dementia. It is committed to the delivery of person-centred, culturally competent care and has considerable experience in working with BAME families.

Ekta
www.ektaproject.org.uk
Based in the London Borough of Newham for the past 30 years, Etka was winner of the Dementia and the Arts Award at the 2015 International Dementia Awards held by Stirling University. The charity has considerable experience in involving arts in dementia awareness-raising.

Irish in Britain
www.irishinbritain.org/what-we-do/our-campaigns/
cuimhne-irish-memory-loss-alliance
Cuimhne – Irish Memory Loss Alliance is a campaign strategy and information resource developed by the organisation Irish in Britain, which covers all aspects of memory loss in later life, including dementia.

Jewish Care
www.jewishcare.org
Jewish Care has a dementia care and support service, based at its Maurice and Vivienne Wohl Campus in North London, which supports those living with dementia and their carers across the whole dementia pathway, from awareness-raising activities to residential care.

Liverpool Dementia Action Alliance
www.youtube.com/channel/UCIdiZ9ZXxcsqbF9ES-96w5Q
The *It's OK to Talk* film project launched in 2015 brought together a number of community groups in Liverpool and built on the role of the existing BAME Dementia Champions funded by Mersey Care NHS Trust. The videos are available on the Dementia Action Alliance YouTube channel.

Meri Yaadain
www.meriyaadain.co.uk
An information and advice service for the South Asian communities in Bradford, established in 2006 by the Council's Adult Services Department.

Nubian Life
www.nubianlife.org.uk
Nubian Life provides adult day care services for older (over 65 years) African and African-Caribbean residents across the London Borough of Hammersmith and Fulham. Its manifesto *Improving Adult Social Care Outcomes and Provision for an Ageing Black and Minority Ethnic & Migrant Population* can be found on the website with a number of other resources.

Pearl Dementia Support Network
www.pearlsupportnetwork.org.uk
The website offers an information resource on services supporting people from BAME communities living with dementia, and information and video material on dementia with a BAME community focus. The support network has done prototyping work to develop a range of reminiscence resources aimed mainly at BAME communities.

Policy Institute for Research on Ageing and Ethnicity
www.priae.org
This organisation was established in 1998 and produced a number of significant documents aimed at the national policy level. Although no longer active, it has produced work on people from Black and minority ethnic elders in long-term care and extra care housing, and its website has an extensive collection of reports on dementia care needs across Europe.

Race Equality Foundation
www.raceequalityfoundation.org.uk
This organisation produces a number of reports on discrimination and disadvantage and is committed to using this knowledge to help overcome barriers and promote race equality in health, housing and social care. The website features several reports on dementia and BAME elders.

Touchstone BME Dementia Team
www.touchstonesupport.org.uk/services/bme-dementia-service
Based in Leeds, the group holds regular awareness-raising sessions in the locality and can hold sessions in English, Punjabi, Hindi and Urdu. It has a regular dementia cafe session called Hamari Yaadain (Our Memories) and has developed important local partnerships to bring the arts into its dementia work.

Author Biographies

Padraic Garrett

Padraic Garrett is a Service Manager with Jewish Care in London. He has worked with staff teams across a wide range of care and community services for over 12 years, upskilling them on person-centred and relationship-focused care. He holds an MSc in Dementia Care from Bradford University. He has a strong interest in the role of community and social networks to support people living with dementia maintain their wellbeing and sense of purpose.

Professor Mark Johnson

Mark R. D. Johnson is Emeritus Professor of Diversity in Health and Social Care at De Montfort University Leicester UK. He founded the Mary Seacole Research Centre and UK Centre for Evidence in Ethnicity, Diversity and Health, the first evidence-based database of research into minority ethnic health issue in Europe. Mark was the first Professor of Diversity in Europe and continues to provide expert advice and input to evaluations, peer reviews, and professional training programmes. He works closely with community members in developing research and policy around issues including dementia. sight loss, musculo-skeletal conditions, learning disability, and health promotion and is passionate about inclusion of people from minority groups in research and development, and communities having access to research evidence.

Dr Karan Jutlla

Dr Karan Jutlla is a a Senior Lecturer in Health (Dementia Lead) for the University of Wolverhampton, UK. Her research and interests in dementia in ethnic minorities has spanned nearly decade. Her doctoral thesis explored how migration experiences impact upon caring for a person with dementia in the Sikh community in Wolverhampton. Karan has since developed education and training to support health care professionals to deliver high quality dementia care for those from South Asian communities. She has undertaken various research projects in this area of work and worked with both private and public organisations to help them meet the dementia challenge for a hitherto neglected but growing part of the community.

Harjinder Kaur

Harjinder Kaur is a retired Community Psychiatric Nurse for Wolverhampton City. In 2001, Harjinder was appointed as the Asian Link nurse with a specialist role to increase contact between specialist old age psychiatry services and older people from South Asian communities in Wolverhampton. Harjinder has played an important role in disseminating information about dementia and related conditions and in educating the South Asian community and professionals on the help available. She is now retired and continues to support elders in the local South Asian communities in accessing help for Mental health problems. She is also a presenter for a local South Asian radio station and has a weekly 'Health is Wealth' programme by way of continuing this education and support.

Tom Lam

Tom Lam was educated at Reading and London School of Economics and has undertaken research projects at the Glyndon Health Project, Greenwich and the Centre for Chinese Studies, South Bank University, on primary healthcare and the Vietnamese in London. He has also taken part in several other research projects on refugee settlement, forced migration, young undocumented chilren and healthcare needs for older Chinese Londoners undertaken at Middlesex University, the City University and Compas (Oxford) and was part of a small team collecting Chinese archival items for the London Metropolitan Archives. He was job-share coordinator for the Chinese Dementia Awareness and Support Project for the Chinese National Healthy Living Centre from 2014–2018. He has published and/or co-authored several articles in healthcare and migration related journals.

Dr Shibley Rahman

Dr Shibley Rahman graduated from Cambridge in medicine, and from London in law and business management. His PhD at Cambridge was in the early diagnosis of behavioural variant frontotemporal dementia. He is also a full-time unpaid family carer, but he maintains a wide range of academic research interests in geriatric medicine and nursing especially dementia, delirium and frailty. He has published widely, including original papers on dementia and books, and he is especially passionate about meaningful person-centred care.

Gill Tan

Gill Tan is a former General/Psychiatric Nurse and Social Worker with a wide-ranging experience in mental health and social work in London and the South East. She was instrumental in setting up the Chinese National Healthy Living Centre and Newham Chinese Association. She has been involved in project development for many years with Chinese community organisations in London to improve mainstream health and care treatment for the Chinese community. Co-working with Tom Lam she ran the Pan-London Chinese Dementia Project at the Chinese National Healthy Living Centre to raise awareness and remove stigma about dementia within the Chinese community.

Dr Mary Tilki

Dr Mary Tilki is a retired university lecturer with professional qualifications in nursing and nursing education. She has researched and published widely on cultural competence in healthcare, ethnic elders, health inequalities and the health of Irish people in Britain. Mary has over twenty years' experience in the UK voluntary sector and has participated in several strategic groups on health inequalities. She has a particular interest in dementia in Irish and other minority ethnic, Gypsy and Traveller communities, especially what culturally sensitive, empowering and inclusive services and care mean for people living with dementia and their family carers.

Natalie Tobert PhD

Dr Natalie Tobert is a Medical Anthropologist, Education Director of Aethos Training. She facilitates participatory workshops on spiritual and cultural awareness for front line staff at hospitals, medical schools, and universities. She co-ordinated the 'Bridging Cultures' project and facilitates mental health promotion events with African and Asian minority ethnic groups in London. Her most recent book Cultural Perspectives on Mental Wellbeing is very well received. Natalie, a Fellow of the Royal Society of Arts, has given conference papers throughout UK, and facilitated retreats and workshops in Poland, Sweden, Switzerland, India, Ireland, Spain and USA.

Social Inclusion website: http://aethos.org.uk

David Truswell

David has worked in community based mental health services in the UK for over thirty years developing services for people with complex care needs and enduring mental health problems in a career spanning the voluntary sector, local authority services, and the NHS at a senior level. From 2009–2011 he was the Dementia Implementation Lead for Commissioning Support for London, working with commissioners across London to improve dementia services. He is currently Executive Director of the Dementia Alliance for Culture and Ethnicity (www.demace.com), a UK social enterprise developed by local and national voluntary organisations working with dementia in Black, Asian and minority ethnic (BAME) communities and is an independent writer and researcher on dementia support and services for BAME communities with a number of journal publications on the issues.

He is also the Director of somefreshthinking limited, a healthcare consultancy working on service redesign and change management in health and social care services.

Toby Williamson

Toby Williamson is an independent consultant working in the fields of adult and older people's mental health, dementia, mental capacity. He also works part time as a lecturer and researcher for the Dementia Care Centre at the University of West London. He has over 30 years' experience working in mental health, managing frontline services, as well as research, training, service development and national policy work. He has recently co-authored 'The Dementia Manifesto', a book on rights, values and dementia published by Cambridge University Press.

Subject Index

Author Index